Intervirology

International Journal of Basic and Medical Virology
Founded 1973 by J.L. Melnick
Continued by F. Rapp (1986–1990)

KARGER

Intervirology
Printed in Switzerland

S. Karger AG,
Postfach, CH – 4009 Basel (Schweiz)

Erscheint zweimonatlich;
pro Jahr 1 Band zu 6 Heften

Intervirology

Submission: Only original papers written in English are considered. Authors should submit the manuscript by air-mail as follows: Original and two copies to the Section Editor of the area in which the paper most suitably fits, with one copy of the submission letter to the Editor-in-Chief; or original and two copies to one of the Editors-in-Chief:

Michael J. Buchmeier
Department of Neuropharmacology
Scripps Clinic and Research Foundation
10666 North Torrey Pines Rd.
La Jolla, CA 92037 (USA)
Phone: 619 554 82 45
FAX-No. 619 554 61 51 (use only for correspondence, not for transmitting manuscripts)

or Colin R. Howard
Department of Clinical Sciences
London School of Hygiene and Tropical Medicine
Keppel Street, London WC1E 7HT (UK)
Phone: 01 636 86 36
FAX-No. 71 636 15 27 (use only for correspondence, not for transmitting manuscripts)

Manuscripts will be reviewed anonymously by Editorial Board members or by other experts in the field. The names of Section Editors and Editorial Board members (by area) are listed on the previous page.

Conditions: All manuscripts are subject to editorial review. Manuscripts are received with the explicit understanding that they are not under simultaneous consideration by any other publication. Submission of an article for publication implies the transfer of the copyright from the author to the publisher upon acceptance. Accepted papers become the permanent property of 'Intervirology' and may not be reproduced by any means, in whole or in part, without the written consent of the publisher. It is the author's responsibility to obtain permission to reproduce illustrations, tables, etc. from other publications.

Arrangement:

Title page: The first page of each paper should indicate the title (main title underlined), the authors' names, and the institute where the work was conducted. A short title for use as a running head is also required.

Key words: For indexing purposes, a list of 3–10 key words in English is essential.

Subject index: The authors should also list 3 or 4 words or brief phrases to be incorporated into the subject index of the volume.

Summary: Each paper needs a summary of up to 10 lines.

Footnotes: Avoid footnotes. When essential, they are numbered consecutively and typed at the foot of the appropriate page.

Body of the paper: Manuscripts should then be divided into the following subdivisions: Introduction, Materials and Methods (as brief as possible), Results, Discussion, Acknowledgments and References.

Tables and illustrations: Tables and illustrations (both numbered in Arabic numerals) should be prepared on separate sheets. Tables require a heading and figures a legend, also prepared on a separate sheet. For the reproduction of illustrations, only good drawings and original photographs can be accepted; negatives or photocopies cannot be used. When possible, group several illustrations on one block for reproduction (max. size 140 × 188 mm) or provide crop marks. On the back of each illustration, indicate its number, the author's name, and 'top'. Color illustrations are reproduced at the author's expense.

References: In the text identify references by Arabic numerals [in square brackets]. Material submitted for publication but not yet accepted should be noted as 'unpublished data' and not be included in the reference list. The list of references should include only those publications which are cited in the text. Do not alphabetize; number references in the order in which they are first mentioned in the text. The surnames of the authors followed by initials should be given. There should be no punctuation other than a comma to separate the authors. Cite all authors, 'et al' is not sufficient. Abbreviate journal names according to the Index Medicus system. (Also see International Committee of Medical Journal Editors: Uniform requirements for manuscripts submitted to biomedical journals. Br Med J 1988;296: 401–405.

Examples

(a) Papers published in periodicals: Kauffman HF, van der Heide S, Beaumont F, Blok H, de Vries K: Class-specific antibody determination against *Aspergillus fumigatus* by means of the enzyme-linked immunosorbent assay. III. Comparative study: IgG, IgA, IgM ELISA titers, precipitating antibodies and IgE binding after fractionation of the antigen. Int Arch Allergy Appl Immunol 1986;80:300–306.

(b) Monographs: Matthews DE, Farewell VT: Using and Understanding Medical Statistics. Basel, Karger, 1985.

(c) Edited books: Hardy WD Jr, Essex M: FeLV-induced feline acquired immune deficiency syndrome: A model for human AIDS; in Klein E (ed): Acquired Immunodeficiency Syndrome. Prog Allergy. Basel, Karger, 1986, vol 37, pp 353–376.

Full address: The exact postal address complete with postal code of the senior author must be given. If correspondence is handled by someone else, indicate this accordingly.

Further details: Authors may consult our leaflet 'Rules for the Preparation of Manuscripts', available on request from the Publisher, S. Karger AG, P.O. Box, CH-4009 Basel (Switzerland).

Nomenclature of viruses: Names used for viruses should be those approved by the International Committee on Taxonomy of Viruses (ICTV) and published in the fourth report of the ICTV 'Classification and Nomenclature of Viruses', Intervirology *17:* 1–200 (1982). If desired, synonyms may be added in parentheses when the name is first mentioned. Approved generic (or group) and family names should also be used.

Short communications: In addition to regular papers, a section of the journal will publish brief communications of important findings, in which illustrative material should be limited. Such notes should include a brief summary and key words, the body of the report (without any subdivisions), brief acknowledgment, and a few selected references. The general style and submission procedures outlined above apply to the short communication.

Commentaries: Short commentaries of an editorial nature may be submitted to the journal. In these communications, usual manuscript subdivisions do not apply, and a summary statement is not needed; however, a very brief reference list may be included.

Page charges: There is no page charge for papers of 8 or fewer printed pages (including tables, illustrations and references). Each additional complete or partial page is charged to the author at SFr. 225.– / US $ 150.00. The allotted size of a paper is equal to approx. 16 manuscript pages (including tables, illustrations and references).

Galley proofs: Unless indicated otherwise, galley proofs are sent to the first-named author and should be returned with the least possible delay. Alterations made in galley proofs, other than the correction of printer's errors, are charged to the author. No page proofs are supplied.

Reprints: Order forms and a price list are sent to the author by the publisher after the article has been set in type. Orders submitted after the issue is printed are subject to considerably higher prices. Allow five weeks from date of publication for delivery of reprints.

Standard forms of abbreviations: The standard abbreviations used for measurements of weight, length, volume, and time (i.e., mg, cm, ml, and min) are acceptable and may be used without definition. The abbreviations listed below also require no preliminary definition. Please note that punctuation is not needed. When using other abbreviations, the name should be spelled out in full at the first mention, and followed with the abbreviation in parentheses.

	degree centigrade (Fahrenheit will not be used)
A, C, G, T, U	adenine, cytosine, guanine, thymine, uracil
AMP	5′-monophosphates of adenosine
CMP	– cytidine
GMP	– guanosine
TMP	– thymidine
UMP	– uridine
ADP, etc.	adenosine 5′-diphosphate, etc.
ATP, etc.	adenosine 5′-triphosphate, etc.
CPE	cytopathic effect
DEAE-cellulose	diethylaminoethylcellulose
DNA	deoxyribonucleic acid
DNase	deoxyribonuclease
EDTA	ethylenediaminetetra-acetate
EOP	efficiency of plating
g	acceleration of gravity
ID_{50}	median infective dose
LD_{50}	median lethal dose
M	molar
MEM	minimum essential medium
MOI	multiplicity of infection
N	normal
ng	nanogram
nm	nanometer (10^{-9} m)
PAGE	polyacrylamide gel electrophoresis
PFU	plaque forming units
RNA	ribonucleic acid
RNase	ribonuclease
rpm	revolutions per minute
SD	standard deviation
SDS	sodium dodecyl sulfate
sp gr	specific gravity
TCD_{50}	median tissue culture infective dose
Tris	tris (hydroxymethyl) aminomethane (2-amino-2-hydroxymethylpropane-1,3-diol)
UV	ultraviolet
V	volt
W	watt

General Information

Publication data: 'Intervirology' is published 6 times annually. Volume 32 with 6 issues appears in 1991.

Subscription rates: Subscriptions run for a full calendar year. Prices are given per volume, surface postage included.

Personal subscription: SFr. 255.50, US$ 167.30 (Must be in the name of, billed to, and paid by an individual. Order must be marked 'personal subscription').

Institutional subscription: SFr. 365.–, US$ 239.00 (Regular rate.)

Members of the International Union of Microbiological Societies, American Association of Immunologists: SFr. 182.50, US$ 119.50.

Airmail postage: SFr. 35.–, US$ 25.00. (Extra per volume.)

Microform subscription: SFr. 182.50, US$ 119.50. (Available exclusively to subscribers of the paper edition.)

Single issues and back volumes: Information on availability and prices can be obtained through the Publisher.

Subscription orders: Orders can be placed at agencies, bookstores, directly with the Publisher S. Karger AG, P.O. Box, CH – 4009 Basel (Switzerland) or with any of the following distributors:

Deutschland, Österreich, Ost-Europa: S. Karger GmbH, Postfach 1724 D – 8034 Germering/München

France: Librairie Luginbühl 36, bd de Latour-Maubourg, F – 75007 Paris

Great Britain, Ireland: S. Karger Publishers, 1 Torberry Drive Petersfield, Hampshire GU 31 4HW

USA: S. Karger Publishers, Inc. 26 West Avon Road, P.O. Box 529 Farmington, CT 06085

India, Bangladesh, Sri Lanka: S. Karger India Subscription Agency B – 5/132 Safdarjung Enclave New Delhi-110029

Japan: Katakura Libri, Inc. 36-9 Hongo 3-chome Bunkyo-ku, Tokyo 113

Change of address: Both old and new address should be stated and sent to the subscription source.

Bibliographic indices: This journal is regularly listed in bibliographic services, including *Current Contents®*.

Advertising: Correspondence and rate requests should be addressed to the Publisher.

KARGER

Vox Sanguinis (ISSN 0042–9007), **Vol. 59, Suppl. 1 (1990)**
Editor: C.P. Engelfriet, Amsterdam

Supplement Issue
Free to journal subscribers

Long-Term Intravenous Immunoglobulin Treatment in Patients with AIDS-Related Complex

Editors: B.A. Perret; P. Imbach, Bern; G.R.F. Krueger, Cologne

This collection of papers presents the results of the first controlled randomized double-blind longitudinal clinical study in which the influence of long-term intravenous immunoglobulin (IVIG) treatment on the clinical status and the T4 cells was evaluated. The study on 30 patients with AIDS-related complex (ARC) and Walter Reed Stage 5 (WR5) showed that the clinical status of patients with advanced HIV infection can be improved by IVIG, although there is little or no influence on the underlying impaired cellular immunity. The issue is of specific interest to those involved in histocompatability oncology, cellular and humoral immunity, complement system and statistics.

Contents

Fields of Interest
Immunology
Infectious Diseases
Hematology

Vox Sanguinis, Vol. 59, Suppl. 1 (1990)
Long-Term Intravenous Immunoglobulin Treatment in Patients with AIDS-Related Complex
Editors: Perret, B.A.; Imbach, P. (Bern); Krueger, G.R.F. (Cologne)
IV + 60 p., 21 fig., 20 tab., soft cover, 1990
SFr. 22.– / DM 26.– / £ 9.60 / US$ 16.50
US$ price for USA, £ price for UK only (subject to change)
ISBN 3–8055–5256–4

KARGER

KI 90195

Latency by Herpes simplex Viruses

Guest Editors:
Kenneth I. Berns, New York, N.Y.
Richard W. Whitley, Birmingham, Ala.

11 figures and 2 tables, 1991

KARGER

S. Karger · Medical and Scientific Publishers
Basel · München · Paris · London · New York · New Delhi · Bangkok · Singapore · Tokyo · Sydney

Drug Dosage

The authors and the publisher have exerted every effort to ensure that drug selection and dosage set forth in this text are in accord with current recommendations and practice at the time of publication. However, in view of ongoing research, changes in government regulations, and the constant flow of information relating to drug therapy and drug reactions, the reader is urged to check the package insert for each drug for any change in indications and dosage and for added warnings and precautions. This is particularly important when the recommended agent is a new and/or infrequently employed drug.

Printed in Switzerland by
Graphische Betriebe Coop Schweiz, Basel
ISBN 3-8055-5362-5

Contents

Intervirology 1991;32:69–75

0300–5526/91/0322–0069$2.75/0

Retention of Nonlinear Viral DNA during Herpes simplex Virus Latency in vitro

Chris M. Preston, Jackie Russell

MRC Virology Unit, Institute of Virology, Glasgow, UK

Key Words. Herpes virus latency · Latent herpes simplex virus · DNA

Summary. We investigated the state of the herpes simplex virus type 2 (HSV-2) genome during latency in vitro. Latent DNA was present in the cell nucleus in a nonlinear configuration. The joint fragment was represented at approximately double the molar concentration of fragments from unique regions, indicating that genome termini had fused. The HSV-2 genome copy number was estimated to be between 1.5 and 8, with a mean value of 4.5 per latently infected cell. Nonlinear HSV DNA can therefore exist during latency both in vivo and in vitro.

Introduction

Herpes simplex virus (HSV) latency involves the prolonged retention of the viral genome in neuronal cells, with occasional reactivation that often results in peripheral lesions. The phenomenon has been reproduced in animal models in which it can, to some extent, be analyzed at a molecular level. Experiments in animals are limited, however, by the low number of cells in sensory ganglia that harbor a potentially active viral genome and the inaccessibility of neurons in situ or after organ culture of ganglia. Tissue culture systems should not suffer from these disadvantages, thus considerable effort has been directed at developing in vitro models that reproduce latency in vivo as faithfully as possible.

We have described an in vitro latency system that is modified from the initial experiments of O'Neill, Rapp and Wigdahl [1–3]. The previous studies showed that suppression of HSV lytic growth by inhibitors of virus replication did not necessarily result in elimination or irreversible inactivation of the viral genome. Infected cultures could be maintained at supraoptimal temperatures of 39.5–40.5° without evidence of active HSV replication, and virus growth always resumed upon downshift to 37°. To establish

Address inquiries to: Dr. C.M. Preston, MRC Virology Unit, Church Street, Glasgow, G11 5JR (UK)

latency, we used incubation at 42° for 6 days rather than the use of inhibitors to suppress the growth of HSV type 2 (HSV-2), and found that, after this treatment, cultures could be returned to 37° without ensuing virus replication [4]. The infectious HSV-2 in the initial inoculum could be recovered, at high efficiency, by superinfection with human cytomegalovirus (HCMV) or with HSV type 1 (HSV-1) temperature-sensitive mutants [4, 5], and subsequent studies demonstrated that the HSV-1 immediate early (IE) protein Vmw110 is responsible for reactivation of latent HSV-2 [5, 6].

There are currently two distinctive properties that characterize the HSV genome during the latent phase. In mouse and human neuronal tissues, terminal DNA fragments cannot be detected and the molecule is thought to be in a nonlinear, possible circular episomal, form [7–10]. Furthermore, only a limited portion of the genome is expressed during latency [11, 12]. Clearly, it would be desirable to demonstrate the occurrence of these two characteristic features in an in vitro latency system, and we report here that one of them, the conversion of the input DNA to a nonlinear form, can be detected in cells infected with HSV-2 at 42°.

Materials and Methods

In vitro Latency

Human fetal lung (HFL) cells were infected with 0.03 PFU of HSV-2 (strain HG52) per cell and incubated at 42°, as described previously [4]. At the time of harvesting, two monolayers were superinfected with 0.001 PFU of HSV-1 *ts*K per cell and incubated at 38.5° for 2 days in the presence of neutralizing human serum [4]. Plaques were counted to provide a measure of the minimum number of cells containing an HSV-2 genome that could be reactivated.

Detection of HSV-2 DNA

HFL cell monolayers were washed twice with ice-cold phosphate-buffered saline, and nuclei prepared as described previously [13]. Nucleic acids were extracted from nuclei as described by Stow et al. [14], and DNA was cleaved by exhaustive digestion with *Bam*HI. Cleaved DNA was mixed with CsCl to give a final volume of 18 ml and a density of 1.708 g/ml, and gradients were formed by centrifugation at 40,000 rpm for 18 h in a Sorvall TV865B vertical rotor. Gradients were fractionated, and fractions representing densities between 1.719 and 1.740 g/ml were pooled. *Escherichia coli* rRNA (20 μg) was added, the pooled fractions were dialyzed against TE (10 mm Tris/HCl, pH 7.5, 1 m*M* EDTA), sodium acetate was added to 0.3 *M*, and nucleic acids were precipitated by the addition of 2.5 vol of ethanol. Precipitates were dissolved in water, incubated with RNase A (100 μg/ml) for 30 min at 25° and electrophoresed on 0.6% agarose gels. DNA fragments were transferred to GeneScreen Plus membranes (NEN), using the capillary blotting method of Southern [15]. Blots were probed with HSV-2 *Bam*HI g or l fragments purified by excision from the pAT153 vector and radiolabeled with ^{32}P by the random primer extension method [16]. Hybridization and washing were performed as described by Park et al. [17], and radiolabeled bands were detected by autoradiography.

Results

Detection of HSV-2 DNA during Latency in vitro

Initial attempts to detect DNA in latently infected cultures by Southern blot hybridization failed because the system can tolerate infection only at relatively low multiplicity. At MOI values above 0.03 PFU of HSV-2 per cell, degeneration of monolayers frequently occurred, and thus the multiplicity required for ready detection of latent DNA (ideally 1 or more PFU per cell) could not be used. In addition, the HSV-2 joint spanning probe, *Bam*HI g, hybridized to cellular DNA resulting in a troublesome background. These problems were overcome by fractionation of latently infected cell DNA on CsCl gradients prior to analysis by hybridization. Fractionated DNA derived from at least 10^7 cells could be run on one lane of an agarose gel, increasing the sensitivity of detection and largely eliminating the problem of hybridization to cellular DNA.

Hybridization of ^{32}P-labeled HSV-2 *Bam*HI g to nuclear DNA from latently infected cells, after incubation at 42° for 4 days, is shown in figure 1. The joint (*Bam*HI g) and termini (*Bam*HI u and v, which comigrate) are clearly visible in a control reconstruction (lane 1) and in a sample of infected cell DNA that was fractionated on a CsCl gradient (lane 5). With DNA from latently infected cells, *Bam*HI g was detected, whereas *Bam*HI u and v were not (lane 2). The HSV-2-specific *Bam*HI g band was distinct from cellular bands that hybridized to the probe (lane 3). Therefore, at 4 days after infection at 42°, nuclear HSV-2 DNA is in a nonlinear conformation.

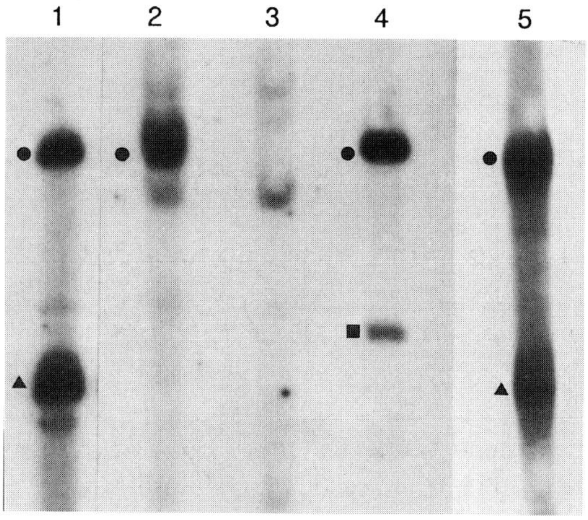

Fig. 1. Nuclear DNA from 3×10^7 cells infected with 0.03 PFU of HSV-2 per cell (lane 2) or mock infected (lane 3) and incubated at 42° for 4 days was banded on CsCl gradients and analyzed by hybridization to radiolabeled HSV-2 *Bam*HI g fragment. Reconstructions containing 1.5×10^7 copies of HSV-2 DNA (lane 1) or cloned *Bam*HI g (lane 4) are also shown. The low level of hybridization to vector pAT153 sequences (■) is due to contamination of the gel-purified *Bam*HI g fragment. DNA from HSV-2-infected HFL cells that was cleaved with *Bam*HI and banded on a CsCl gradient is shown (lane 5). The positions of joint (*Bam*HI g, ●) and terminal (*Bam*HI u and v, ▲) fragments are indicated.

Molarity of the Bam*HI g Fragment*

As discussed by Rock and Fraser [8], the absence of termini could be due to circularization, concatemerization or integration of the latent genome. Circularization, concatemerization or integration via internal U_L or U_S regions of the genome would yield a joint fragment that is 2 *M* with respect to a fragment from a unique region of the genome, whereas random integration via the termini would result in heterogeneous, novel terminal fragments and a joint remaining at 1 *M*. DNA from latently infected cells was therefore probed with a mixture of ^{32}P-labeled *Bam*HI g and *Bam*HI l and the relative intensities of hybridization determined by densitometry. An example of a result from this experiment is shown in figure 2: by observation, it is clear that for DNA from latently infected cells (lane 1) hybridization to *Bam*HI g is more intense, relative to *Bam*HI l, than in the reconstructions (lanes 3 and 4). In 5 repetitions of this procedure, after correcting the intensities of the *Bam*HI g and *Bam*HI l signals to a relative value of 1 in the reconstructions, the molarity of *Bam*HI g was found to vary between 1.4 and 2.4, with a mean value of 1.85. It appears, therefore, that HSV-2 DNA during latency in vitro is predominantly either circular, concatemeric or integrated via regions other than the genome termini.

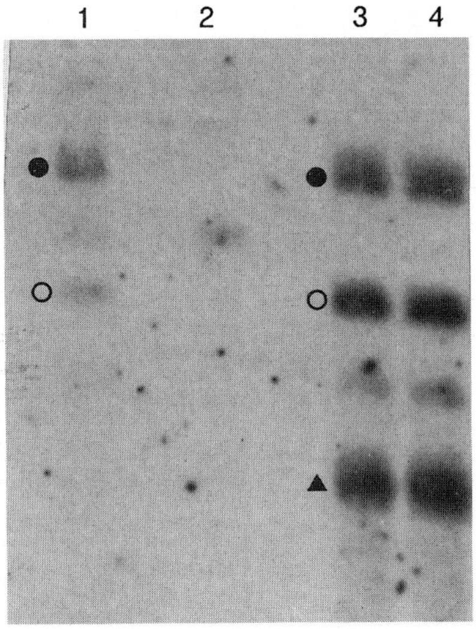

Fig. 2. Nuclear DNA from 2×10^7 cells infected with 0.03 PFU of HSV-2 per cell (lane 1) or mock infected (lane 2) and incubated at 42° for 4 days was banded on CsCl gradients and analyzed by hybridization to a mixture of radiolabeled HSV-2 *Bam*HI g and l fragments. Reconstructions contained 3×10^6 (lane 3) or 10^7 (lane 4) copies of HSV-2 DNA. The positions of joint (*Bam*HI g, ●), unique (*Bam*HI l, ○) and terminal (*Bam*HI u and v, ▲) fragments are shown.

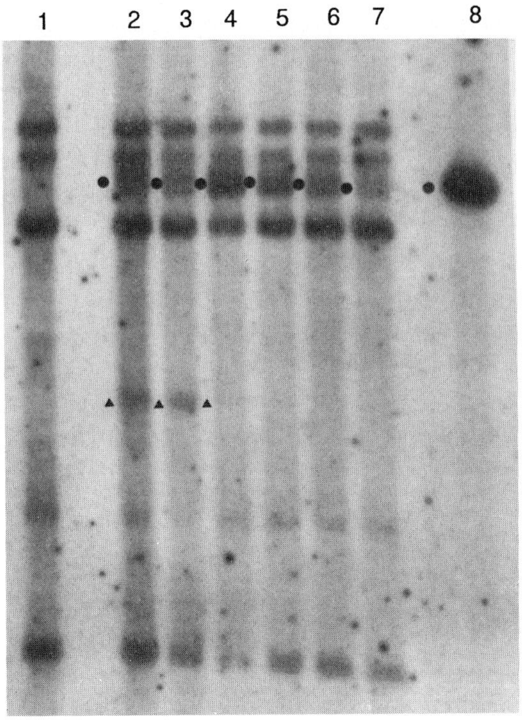

Fig. 3. Cells were mock infected (lane 1) or infected with 0.03 PFU of HSV-2 per cell and incubated at 42° for 1 (lane 2), 2 (lane 3), 3 (lane 4), 4 (lane 5), 5 (lane 6) or 6 (lane 7) days. Nuclear DNA from 1.8×10^7 cells was banded on CsCl gradients and analyzed by hybridization to radiolabeled HSV-2 *Bam*HI g. A sample containing 1.5×10^7 copies of cloned *Bam*HI g is also shown (lane;8), and the positions of joint (*Bam*HI g, ●) and terminal (*Bam*HI u and v, ▲) fragments are indicated.

Conversion to Nonlinear DNA Occurs Slowly

Nuclear DNA in HSV-2-infected cells was examined during incubation at 42° (fig. 3). After 1 day, termini and joint fragments were represented (lane 2). Hybridization to terminal fragments decreased during days 2 and 3 (lanes 3 and 4) and was undetectable by day 4 (lane 5). During this period, hybridization to the joint fragment *Bam*HI g was apparent at relatively constant levels, although the signal became weaker by day 6 (lane 7). Thus, conversion of HSV-2 DNA to the nonlinear state occurred slowly, over a 4-day period. The presence of two *Bam*HI g bands in this experiment is probably due to differences in the number of 'a' sequences.

Quantitation of Latent DNA

Two methods are available to estimate the amount of viral DNA present in latently infected cultures. Upon superinfection with 0.001 PFU of *ts*K per cell, between 50 and 120

PFU were reactivated from cultures of 3×10^6 cells initially infected with 10^5 PFU of HSV-2, suggesting that between 5×10^4 and 1.2×10^5 PFU (about 100% of the PFU initially applied to the HFL cell cultures) could be recovered. Thus, at least 10^5 genomes are present per 3×10^6 cells. However, calculation of the amount of HSV-2 DNA from the intensity of the hybridization signal, compared with reconstructions, gives a mean value of 4.5×10^5 genomes per 3×10^6 cells, with a range of 1.5×10^5 to 8.0×10^5. Therefore, extensive replication of the input genome does not occur at 42°, as suggested by the data in figure 3 and previous reports [18, 19], but a proportion of the genomes detected by hybridization may not be competent for reactivation by superinfection with *ts*K.

Discussion

We report here the first demonstration that nonlinear HSV DNA can be maintained in an in vitro latency system. The observation substantiates our belief that the in vitro model reproduces at least some aspects of latency in vivo and can therefore give relevant information. The use of CsCl banding to enrich for HSV-2 sequences increased the sensitivity of detection to a level at which viral DNA can be identified even after initial infection at 0.03 PFU per cell. No *Bam*HI g-specific hybridization was detected when cytoplasmic fractions were analyzed [J.R., unpubl. results], suggesting that the HSV-2 DNA persisting in the cultures was confined to the nucleus. The relatively slow conversion of HSV-2 DNA to a nonlinear form suggests a process that is different from the rapid fusion of termini reported to occur after infection under permissive conditions [20].

In mouse model systems of latency, the number of genomes detected far exceeds the number of neuronal cells estimated to contain virus that can be reactivated by explant [9, 21, 22]. Thus, either many more cells harbor latent HSV than can be detected by explant, or the viral genome is present in hundreds of copies per latently infected neuron. It is not possible, therefore, to determine whether the nonlinear DNA represents potentially active genomes or a population of molecules that can never be reactivated. With the in vitro system, although a precise copy number per latently infected cell is also difficult to obtain due to the accumulation of errors during calculations, the excess of genomes over reactivatable viruses is not greater than 8-fold. Since termini could be detected if they were present at 8-fold lower concentration than the joint fragment (fig. 1), it is clear that at least some of the nonlinear molecules can give rise to infectious virus upon reactivation. It will be interesting to determine whether the genome remains nonlinear or is converted back to a linear form during reactivation.

Although our in vitro latency system is similar to that of Wigdahl et al. [3], in which virus replication is initially suppressed by treatment with interferon and 5-(2-bromovinyl)-2′-deoxyuridine, an increasing number of differences are becoming apparent. As pointed out by Scheck et al. [23], reactivation in 'inhibitor-induced' latency requires more than the presence of HSV IE proteins, whereas in our '42°-induced' system the HSV-1 IE protein Vmw110 is the sole requirement for reactivation [5, 6]. Reactivation in the inhibitor-induced system always occurs upon temperature downshift to 37° [2] and can be accelerated by induction of cellular DNA synthesis [24], whereas the 42°-induced system is stable in the short term, even after subculture and reseeding of monolayers at 37° [4]. Finally, latent DNA is predominantly linear in the inhibitor-induced system [25] but nonlinear in 42°-treated cells. From these comparisons, the two systems appear to be fundamentally different. A rationalization may be found in the work of Shiraki and Rapp [26], which suggested that two populations of cells harboring HSV exist during inhibitor-induced latency. One population was reactivated upon temperature downshift to 37° while the other required superinfection with HCMV for reactivation. Perhaps the latter population resembles the 42°-induced latency system.

The maintenance of HSV DNA in a nonlinear form, resembling that found during latency in vivo, is an encouraging indicator that the in vitro latency system can provide relevant information. Future studies can now focus on details of the structure and expression of the latent genome.

Acknowledgments

We thank Prof. J.H. Subak-Sharpe for his interest in this work. J.R. was supported by a Medical Research Council Research Training Award.

References

1 O'Neill FJ: Prolongation of herpes simplex virus latency in cultured human cells by temperature elevation. J Virol 1977;24:41–46.
2 Wigdahl BL, Isom HC, Rapp F: Repression and activation of the genome of herpes simplex viruses in human cells. Proc Natl Acad Sci USA 1981; 78:6522–6526.
3 Wigdahl BL, Scheck AC, DeClercq E, et al: High efficiency latency and activation of herpes simplex virus in human cells. Science 1982;217: 1145–1146.
4 Russell J, Preston CM: An in vitro latency system for herpes simplex virus type 2. J Gen Virol 1986; 67:397–403.
5 Russell J, Stow ND, Stow EC, et al: Herpes simplex virus genes involved in latency in vitro. J Gen Virol 1987;68:3009–3018.
6 Harris RA, Everett RD, Zhu X, et al: Herpes simplex virus type 1 immediate early protein Vmw110 reactivates latent herpes simplex virus type 2 in an in vitro latency system. J Virol 1989;63:3513–3515.
7 Rock DL, Fraser NW: Detection of HSV-1 genome in the central nervous system of latently infected mice. Nature 1983;302:523–525.
8 Rock DL, Fraser, NW: Latent herpes simplex virus type 1 DNA contains two copies of the virion DNA joint region. J Virol 1985;55:849–852.
9 Efstathiou S, Minson AC, Field HJ, et al: Detection of herpes simplex virus-specific DNA sequences in latently infected mice and in humans. J Virol 1986;57:446–455.
10 Mellerick DM, Fraser NW: Physical state of the latent herpes simplex virus genome in a mouse model system: Evidence suggesting an episomal state. Virology 1987;158:265–275.
11 Stevens JG, Wagner EK, Devi-Rao GB, et al: RNA complementary to a herpesvirus alpha gene mRNA is prominent in latently infected neurons. Science 1987;235:1056–1059.
12 Spivack JG, Fraser NW: Detection of herpes simplex virus type 1 transcripts during latent infection in mice. J Virol 1987;61:3841–3847.
13 Preston CM: Abnormal properties of an immediate early polypeptide in cells infected with the herpes simplex virus type 1 mutant tsK. J Virol 1979;32:357–369.
14 Stow ND, Murray MD, Stow EC: Cis-acting signals involved in the replication and packaging of herpes simplex virus type 1 DNA; in Botchan M, Grodzicker T, Sharp PA (eds): Cancer Cells. DNA Tumour Viruses: Control of Gene Expression and Replication. Cold Spring Harbor, Cold Spring Harbor Laboratory, 1986, vol 4, pp 497–507.
15 Southern EM: Detection of specific sequences among DNA fragments separated by gel electrophoresis. J Mol Biol 1975;98:503–517.
16 Feinberg AP, Vogelstein B: A technique for radi-

olabeling DNA restriction endonuclease fragments to high specific activity. Anal Biochem 1983;132:6–13.

17 Park M, Kitchener HC, Macnab JCM: Detection of herpes simplex virus type-2 DNA restriction fragments in human cervical carcinoma tissue, EMBO J 1983;2:1029–1034.

18 Crouch NA, Rapp F: Cell-dependent differences in the production of infectious herpes simplex virus at a supraoptimal temperature. J Virol 1972;9:223–230.

19 Marcon MJ, Kucera LS: Consequences of herpes simplex virus type 2 and human cell interaction at supraoptimal temperatures. J Virol 1976;20: 54–62.

20 Poffenberger KL, Roizman B: A noninverting genome of a viable herpes simplex virus 1: Presence of head-to-tail linkages in packaged genomes and requirements for circularization after infection. J Virol 1985;53:587–595.

21 Cabrera CV, Wohlenberg C, Openshaw H, et al: Herpes simplex virus DNA sequences in the CNS of latently infected mice. Nature 1980;288: 288–290.

22 Roizman B, Sears AE: An inquiry into the mechanisms of herpes simplex virus latency. Ann Rev Microbiol 1987;41:543–571.

23 Scheck AC, Wigdahl B, Rapp F: Activation of latent herpes simplex virus type 2 infection in vitro requires a (E)-5-(2-bromovinyl)-2′-deoxyuridine-sensitive gene function. Intervirology 1987;27: 121–129.

24 Vonka V, Shiraki K, Wrzos J, et al: Cellular DNA synthesis associated with activation of latent herpes simplex virus in cell culture. Intervirology 1986;25:144–150.

25 Wigdahl B, Scheck AC, Ziegler RJ, et al: Analysis of the herpes simplex virus genome during in vitro latency in human diploid fibroblasts and rat sensory neurons. J Virol 1984;49:205–213.

26 Shiraki K, Rapp F: Establishment of herpes simplex virus latency in vitro with cycloheximide. J Gen Virol 1986;67:2497–2500.

Intervirology 1991;32:76–92

0300–5526/91/0322–0076$2.75/0

Role of Herpes simplex Virus Thymidine Kinase Expression in Viral Pathogenesis and Latency

Richard B. Tenser

Department of Medicine (Neurology), and Microbiology and Immunology, Pennsylvania State University College of Medicine, Hershey, Pa., USA

Key Words. Thymidine kinase · Latent infection

Summary. Herpes simplex virus (HSV) thymidine kinase (TK) expression and the HSV TK gene have been evaluated in studies of gene control, as well as in animal and human studies of viral pathogenesis, including HSV latency. In investigations of the biological role of HSV TK, enzyme expression was noted to be important for HSV infection of nonreplicating cells in culture; and, in experimental animal studies, HSV TK was shown to be important for in vivo latent infection of sensory ganglion neurons. Latency in these studies was determined by the ability of HSV to reactivate from sensory ganglion explants. In recent studies, investigators sought to determine whether the role HSV TK expression plays in latency is primarily in the establishment and maintenance of latency or in the reactivation process. Following infection of experimental animals with HSV TK-deficient mutants, the presence of HSV in ganglia was detected in complementation, rescue, and molecular biological studies. Results suggest that HSV TK expression may be important for HSV reactivation from latency. This was supported by in situ hybridization investigations. In the latter studies, HSV latency associated transcript (LAT) was present in ganglion neurons, although reactivation of HSV from such ganglia was defective. LAT-expressing, reactivation-defective infections established by TK mutants of HSV are considered examples of incomplete latency. From the present review, it appears that HSV TK expression, particularly TK expression of HSV-1, is important for the reactivation of latent HSV infection of sensory ganglion neurons, probably because of limited neuronal TK expression and absent replication capacity of these cells.

Introduction

In 1963, the induction of thymidine kinase (TK) enzyme activity in herpes simplex virus (HSV)-infected cells was reported by Kit and Dubbs [1], and similar results were reported

Address inquiries to: Dr. Richard B. Tenser, Division of Neurology, Pennsylvania State University College of Medicine, 500 University Drive, Hershey, PA 17033 (USA)

in pseudorabies virus-infected cells by Nohara and Kaplan [2]. The latter publication was the first to report that the TK activity induced by the herpesvirus infection was virus specific [2], and within several years, it was evident that HSV expressed viral-specific TK activity [3–6]. Over the ensuing years, TK genes and TK enzyme activity were described for many herpesviruses (table 1), as well as other DNA viruses [27, 28]; and, it is expected that viral-specific TK activity will be reported for other viruses, including other herpesviruses. HSV TK, particularly that of HSV-type 1 (HSV-1), was intensively investigated and will be emphasized in this report.

The HSV TK gene is used as a marker in studies of the biochemical transformation of TK-deficient cells [29-32]; and, such studies provided the impetus for determinations of the genetic localization (at approximately 0.3 map units) of the HSV-1 and HSV-2 TK genes [33–36] and also the sequencing of the HSV TK genes [37–41]. Recent studies have investigated the effect of methylation of the HSV TK gene on gene expression [42, 43]. Information gained in early investigations permitted molecular biological studies in which the HSV TK gene was utilized as a model for the analysis of genetic control and expression [44–47]. In other molecular studies, specific insertions and deletions were incorporated into the HSV genome as a means of introducing genetic information into the HSV genome and to construct TK-deficient mutants [48–52]. Most recently, transgenic mice carrying the HSV TK gene were created [53, 54].

In polyacrylamide gel studies, HSV TK is reported to have a molecular weight in the denatured form of 40,00–45,000 daltons [55, 56] and approximately 82,000 daltons [57] in the nondenatured biologically active dimer form. Recently, HSV TK was purified and crystallized [58]. It was noted that HSV TK possessed thymidylate kinase activity [59, 60], and unlike cellular TKs readily phosphorylated various pyrimidine deoxynucleotides [61–64]. This promiscuous behavior by HSV TK was important in the development of specific antivirals such as acyclovir, since this drug is phosphorylated to the active antiviral form by HSV TK [65–67]. Biochemical aspects of HSV TK were recently reviewed by Kit [68].

Table 1. Herpesviruses with identified tk genes and viral TK activity

Virus
Human herpesviruses
HSV-1 [3–5]
HSV-2 [6, 7]
Varicella zoster virus [8–10]
Epstein-Barr virus [11–13]
Animal herpesviruses
Pseudorabies virus [2, 14]
Equine herpesvirus type 1 [15]
Equine herpesvirus type 3 [16]
Bovine herpesvirus type 1 [17, 18]
Bovine herpesvirus type 2 [19]
Bovine herpesvirus type 4 [20]
Herpesvirus of turkeys [21, 22]
Marek's disease virus [23]
Feline herpesvirus [24]
Marmoset herpesvirus (tamarinus) [25]
Herpesvirus saimiri [26]
Herpesvirus ateles [26]

Biological functions of HSV TK were not initially evident, and in early studies it is noted that HSV TK expression is not generally important for viral infection in cell culture [3]. The first suggestion of a possible biological role for HSV TK was in 1974 when Jamieson et al. [62] reported that, although

HSV TK expression is dispensable for HSV infection of dividing cells in culture, TK expression is important for infection of nondividing cells. We pursued our subsequent investigations of the role of HSV TK expression in in vivo latent infection for this reason, and because HSV latency was considered to be an infection of nondividing neurons.

Initial in vivo use of presumptive HSV TK mutants was reported in 1975 by Marcialis at al. [69] who noted that iododeoxyuridine-resistant HSV-1 mutants were much less virulent in mice and rabbits than were the parental viruses. In addition, infection of animals with these mutants protected against subsequent challenge with parental HSV, probably due to immunization by the former. HSV mutants were probably TK deficient, but no mention of viral TK activity was made. Several years later Field and Wildy [70] and Tenser and co-workers [71, 72] investigated neurovirulence and HSV latent infection after inoculation of mice and guinea pigs with HSV TK mutants. Since then, several reports note a decreased neurovirulence, i.e. decreased mortality after animal inoculation with many different HSV TK mutants [73–79]. There have been exceptions to this trend [80, 81], however, and virulent HSV TK mutants are of potential importance in a more complete understanding of HSV neurovirulence. Decreased virulence also was noted with TK mutants of pseudorabies virus [13, 82, 83]. Neurovirulence may bear a relationship to latency, at least to the extent that if a virus is too virulent, the host will succumb and latency will not be measurable, although the relationship may be more direct as common viral or cellular factors may be involved. At the present time, however, they will be considered separate entities, and the remainder of this report will focus on latency.

Latency

Before further discussion of HSV TK expression and latency, it is necessary to consider the operational definition of latency and to describe the experimental procedures used to investigate HSV latency. Investigators generally have inoculated experimental animals (mice, guinea pigs, rabbits) with HSV after scarification or other traumatization at the site of inoculation. Inoculation has been at a site innervated by peripheral axons of sensory ganglion neurons, less commonly a site innervated by autonomic ganglion or motor neurons. The site of inoculation is distal to the ganglion tissue to be studied, and the procedure most often assumes local replication of the virus at the site of inoculation followed by retrograde axoplasmic transport of virus to ganglion neurons. The ganglion is acutely infected by this process and some neurons are probably destroyed, while a latent and nondestructive infection is established in others.

At the outset we will consider HSV latency to be a long-term infection, best identified in neurons, which is largely inapparent, resulting in the reactivation of infectious HSV after explant culture. The isolation of infectious HSV after explant culture of latently infected ganglia, but not from ganglion homogenates, was the primary operational criterion established by Stevens and co-workers [84, 85], and it suggests the presence of HSV in an incomplete form. It also suggests the requirement of a cellular contribution to the reactivation process, which results in the synthesis of infectious HSV. Animal models of HSV latency approximate, but possibly do not always duplicate, human HSV latency and in vivo reactivation in humans. Similarities and difference between in vivo reactivation and in vitro reactivation in ganglion tissue explants will not be pursued here. As noted later in discussions of recent investigations of HSV TK mutants, the definition of HSV latency, vis-à-vis reactivation in infectious virus, will partially determine how biological function is ascribed to HSV TK expression.

The last housekeeping issue to consider pertains to the TK phenotype of HSV TK mutants with which experimental animals are inoculated. This is necessary since (i) mutations may result in varying degrees of TK expression [56, 75, 86–89], and (ii) intermediate levels of HSV TK expression may be sufficient for significant acute infection and for latency [77, 90–93]. The issue is further complicated because of the occurrence of mixtures of infectious HSV particles which express varying levels of TK activity. Via TK complementation, this may result in pathogenesis and latency of TK mutants when more pure populations of TK negative (TK^-) HSV do not [91–93]. Interallelic complementation between HSV TK mutants in cell culture was reported by Jamieson and Subak-Sharpe [94] and is predicated on the active TK enzyme being a dimer, and also the occurrence of TK mutants with defects at different sites. It is also necessary to consider the TK phenotype of HSV isolated during latency, as well as virus inoculated, because of complementation and because of possible reversion, particularly if nondeletion mutants are used for animal inoculations.

Several assays of TK activity are utilized to determine the TK phenotype of HSV, including cell-free phosphorylation of thymidine and other nucleotides [31, 95, 96], sensitivity of HSV replication to antivirals which require HSV TK expression for their activation [65, 66, 87, 97, 98], and thymidine plaque autoradiography [88, 89, 99, 100]. The first

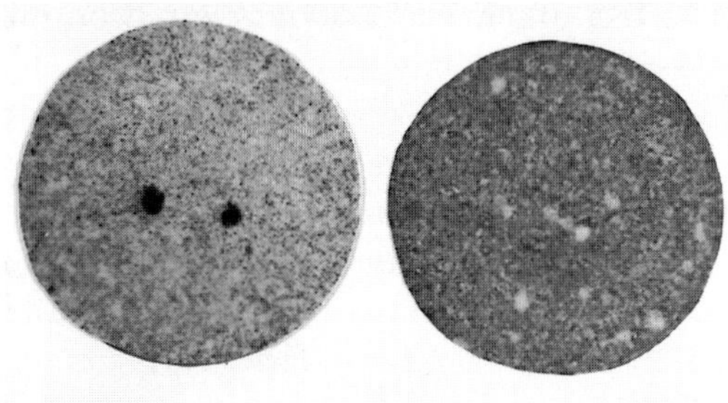

Fig. 1. HSV-1 TK phenotype determined by plaque autoradiography. Left: Rabbit kidney cell monolayer culture infected with TK^+ and TK^- HSV, showing 17 HSV plaques. Right: Autoradiography of this culture showing that 2 of the plaques are TK^+ HSV. The monolayer culture was incubated with medium containing [^{14}C]thymidine (0.5 μCi/ml) for 5 h. After washing and fixation, the dried monolayer was placed in contact with X-ray film for 5 days [89, 100].

two types of assays are useful in testing large populations of HSV and are relatively insensitive to the presence of mixtures of TK^+ and TK^- HSV, particularly mixtures with small amounts of HSV of one or the other TK phenotypes. Plaque autoradiography is a qualitative assay of individual HSV plaques, and is useful to identify mixtures of TK^+ and TK^- HSV. It is particularly valuable for identification of the TK phenotype of HSV isolated from latently infected tissues. The plaque autoradiography procedure reflects viral TK activity expressed over several hours in infected cells, and may be more biologically relevant at times than a briefer biochemical assay of cell-free enzyme activity. An example of HSV plaque autoradiography is seen in figure 1.

We have generally utilized thymidine phosphorylation assay on HSV stocks, and have utilized plaque autoradiography assays on HSV stocks and on animal isolates. The value of appropriate TK assays cannot be minimized, since the attribution of a biological effect of TK expression is based on the measured TK phenotype. We have generally considered TK⁻ HSV to refer to HSV which expresses <5% of parental TK activity and is TK⁻ by plaque autoradiographic assay. The term HSV TK mutant is used to refer to similar mutants but also to HSV mutants with less clearly determined or less clearly limited TK activity.

Role of HSV TK Expression in Latency

Detection of Infectious Virus

In 1978, Field and Wildy [70] noted decreased ganglion latency after inoculation of mice with TK⁻ mutants of HSV-1 and HSV-2. Their emphasis was on virus virulence, and their view of the role of HSV TK expression in latency was somewhat equivocal, as indicated by their conclusion that TK⁻ mutant virus is able to establish latency despite the enzyme deficiency. Alternatively, they may have been prescient in their conclusion and anticipated recent reports of the role of HSV TK in latency, which depend in part on definitions of latency. This will be discussed in detail below.

In 1979, we reported decreased trigeminal ganglion latency in guinea pigs [71] and in mice [72] after corneal inoculation with either of the two HSV-1 TK⁻ mutants. Since both TK mutants replicated well in the cornea – a site of replicating or potentially replicating cells, but latency was decreased in the sensory ganglion (neurons) – we suggest that HSV TK expression is important for neuronal infection and latency [72]. As noted above, this was potentially anticipated by the report of Jamieson et al. [62] that HSV TK expression was not important for infection of replicating cells but was important for those not replicating. Additional in vivo support for this conclusion was found in studies of TK⁻ HSV replication in the liver of mice with and without prior partial hepatectomy, which procedure results in the rapid in vivo replication of liver cells [101].

It should be emphasized that in the studies of Field and Wildy [70] and Tenser and co-worker [71, 72], the presence of latency was determined by the reactivation of HSV from explanted ganglia. This was in keeping with many prior investigations of HSV latency and the general concept of HSV latency previously established [84, 85].

In these initial studies, it was noted that in addition to decreased HSV latency, inoculation of mice with TK⁻ HSV resulted in decreased HSV replication in ganglia during the acute period of infection (days 2–5 post-inoculation) [71, 72]. It was, in part, for this reason that we hypothesized that HSV TK had an important role in the establishment of latency (i.e. infection with TK mutants resulted in decreased HSV replication during the acute infection and this resulted in decreased latency). HSV replication at the site of inoculation is important, at least to ensure an adequate viral inoculum. However, a requirement for HSV and/or HSV DNA replication in ganglion neurons during the establishment of latency is without supportive evidence. In fact, evidence has been reported that such replication during the establishment of latency need not occur [102–104]. At the time of our early studies, it was suggested by others that, rather than being important for the establishment of latency, HSV TK may be important for viral reactivation [Price, personal commun.]; as will be seen later, this is probably correct.

Following the initial studies by Field and Wildy [70] and Tenser and co-workers [71,

72], several investigators reported results which supported an important role for HSV TK expression in HSV latency [50, 73–75, 77, 78], including an investigation of in vitro infection of ganglion neurons [105]. A few studies, however, suggested a lesser or unimportant role [106–110]. The latter group of studies included one in which the investigators studied HSV-2 [107] which is often of increased virulence and may have a lesser dependence on TK expression [78], and another in which immunosuppression appeared to heighten latency following HSV TK mutant infection [106]. In another study, it appeared that there might be a lesser role for HSV TK expression in an animal species such as the rabbit [109]. This observation may be of importance in indicating biological diversity, including, for example, the possibility that complementation of TK^- HSV by cellular TK occurred with some frequency in this species, and, therefore, may have diminished the necessity for expression of the viral enzyme. It also remains possible that TK^- HSV may establish latent infection if activity of other viral or cellular functions compensated for diminished HSV TK activity. For example, we found that age may be a factor. After corneal inoculation of adult mice with some HSV TK^- mutants, we noted reactivation of HSV from trigeminal ganglia in up to 6%, while reactivation occurred in 20% when mice were inoculated as newborns [unpubl. data].

When considering studies which minimize the role of HSV TK expression in latency, it is also important to (i) determine whether there is sufficient TK characterization of HSV mutants used [88], since mutants which are not sufficiently TK defective, may replicate in ganglia to varying levels [87], and may establish latent infections [75, 77, 90–92], and (ii) determine whether TK^+ HSV is present in the TK^- HSV stock used, since this may result in TK complementation.

TK complementation between TK mutants was reported in cell culture as the result of interallelic complementation [94]. In animal studies, TK complementation between TK mutants and by TK^+ HSV resulted in acute TK^- HSV infection and TK^- HSV latency, after the inoculation of mixtures of TK^+ and TK^- HSV [87, 91–93]. The clinical development of mixtures of TK^+ and TK^- may occur following the treatment of immunosuppressed patients with medications like acyclovir, and it is anticipated that this may result in HSV TK complementation in humans. Per se, the occurrence of TK complementation supports an important role for HSV TK expression in latency and pathogenesis. It should be noted that, although most HSV TK mutants are resistant to acyclovir because of limited or absent TK expression, including those isolated from immunosuppressed acyclovir-treated patients [110–112], other mutants may be resistant to acyclovir because of altered enzyme substrate specificity [75, 96, 113, 114] or altered HSV DNA polymerase [114–116]. The latter two types of mutants are expected to be acyclovir resistant but TK^+ (thymidine phosphorylation positive), and it is concluded that TK phenotype and acyclovir sensitivity should be considered separately. It may also be noted that HSV TKs are abnormal in other ways, including temperature sensitivity, sensitivity to salt concentration, and ATP (phosphate donor) binding [96, 117, 118]. These factors may be important in biological systems and may be necessary to take into account in assays to determine the TK phenotype of HSV TK mutants (table 2).

In recent years, investigations with defined HSV TK deletion mutants have further

Table 2. Characteristics of HSV-1 TK and infection with TK mutants

Property or characteristic
Gene site at 0.3 map units [33–35]
Molecular weight of
Denatured form, 40,000–45,000 daltons [55, 56]
Biologically active dimer form, 82,000 daltons [57]
Biochemical transformation of TK⁻ cells [29–33]
Phosphorylation of multiple nucleotides [61–67]
Phosphorylation of thymidylate [59, 60]
Important for HSV replication in nondividing cells [62, 70]
Development of TK⁻ HSV mutants in patients [110–112]
Construction of TK⁻ HSV deletion mutants [50–52, 92]
Assays of HSV TK activity by
Thymidine phosphorylation [29, 95, 96]
Drug inhibition [65, 66, 87, 97, 98]
Plaque autoradiography [88, 89, 99, 100]
Poor isolation of TK⁻ HSV from sensory ganglia [70–78]
Complementation of TK⁻ HSV by TK⁺ HSV in sensory ganglia [91–93]
Expression of TK⁻ HSV gene products in sensory ganglia [50, 51, 119, 128]
Rescue of TK⁻ HSV from sensory ganglia [50, 51]

supported an important role of HSV TK expression in latency [50–52, 92], and the present emphasis is on where in the establishment-of-latency-reactivation sequence of events is HSV TK expression important. Specifically, investigators have sought to determine whether HSV TK expression is important in the establishment or maintenance of latency or whether it is important in the reactivation process.

In a clever molecular biological study, Ho and Mocarski [119] show that after peripheral inoculation of mice with TK⁻ HSV, evidence of the virus could be detected in ganglion neurons. In this study, β-galactosidase expression was detected in ganglia after inoculation of TK⁻ HSV in which the *Escherichia coli* lacZ gene was inserted into the HSV genome and placed under control of viral regulatory signals. This study provided evidence of viral gene expression in ganglion neurons after inoculation of TK⁻ HSV, although infectious virus was not isolated from ganglia [119]. In related preliminary studies, we occasionally could detect HSV antigen during the period of acute infection after inoculation of TK⁻ HSV, including testing with a monoclonal antibody to infected cell polypeptide 4 (ICP 4) [unpublished data]. More definitive evidence of the presence of TK⁻ HSV in ganglion tissue was provided by two studies in which it was demonstrated that during latency infectious TK⁻ HSV could be rescued from ganglion tissues by in vitro superinfection of the tissues [50, 51] (table 2).

In an in vivo complementation study, further evidence of the presence of TK⁻ HSV in ganglia during latency is provided, and it appeared that TK⁻ and TK⁺ HSV genomes were present in the same neurons [92]. In this study, inoculation of mice with TK⁻ HSV alone resulted in a lack of reactivatable HSV during latency, while inoculation of TK⁻ – TK⁺ HSV mixtures resulted in the isolation of TK⁻ and TK⁺ HSV during latency. Reactivation of latently infected ganglion explants cultured in medium containing arabinosylthymine (ara-T) resulted in the expected absence of detectable TK⁺ HSV but also the absence of detectable TK⁻ HSV. The inhibitory effect of ara-T on the reactivation and isolation of TK⁻ HSV suggests that: (i) ara-T was phosphorylated by TK⁺ HSV to the active antiviral and then inhibited TK⁺ and

TK⁻ HSV DNA polymerase, or (ii) only TK⁺ HSV was inhibited, with the result that TK complementation and reactivation of TK⁻ HSV did not occur. The latter possibility suggests a role for HSV TK expression in the reactivation process. Both explantations are most consistent with TK⁻ HSV being in cells which also contain TK⁺ HSV.

These groups of studies suggest that after inoculation with TK⁻ HSV, mutant virus is present in sensory ganglia, probably in ganglion neurons. Although TK⁻ HSV usually does not reactivate from ganglion explants when inoculated alone, under some circumstances infectious TK⁻ HSV is recovered. From this information, it appears that TK⁻ HSV is present in ganglia for extended periods of time, and depending on definitions of HSV latency, it could be argued that TK⁻ HSV established latent infections.

Detection of Virus-Specified RNA

A recent group of investigations of latency with TK⁻ HSV mutants has utilized in situ and blot hybridization in order to study, more extensively, the nature of in vivo TK⁻ HSV infection of the sensory ganglion neurons. These studies followed the initial use of purified HSV DNA for the in situ hybridization detection of HSV-specified RNA [120, 121]. In the more recent hybridization investigations, cloned HSV DNA fragments were used to determine specific HSV RNA species present during latency [122–126]. In this group of studies, Stevens et al. [122], and then other investigators [122–127], reported that hybridization was detected with only specifically cloned fragments and with only one DNA strand of the fragments. Several investigators have identified 2–3 specific RNA species transcribed during latency. HSV latency-associated transcripts (LAT) are extensively discussed elsewhere in this publication by Nsiah and Rapp. In recent studies, investigators have investigated whether LAT is present in sensory ganglia after TK⁻ HSV infection.

In 1989, three groups reported the presence of LAT in ganglion neurons by in situ hybridization following inoculation of mice with TK⁻ HSV-1 [51, 52, 128]. LAT hybridization in ganglia latently infected by TK⁻ HSV-1 is seen in figure 2; hybridization by a cloned DNA probe and by a synthetic oligonucleotide probe are seen. Detection of LAT in sensory ganglia after inoculation of TK⁻ HSV-2 has also been noted [unpubl. data]. In a quantitative study, the number of LAT-expressing neurons after TK⁻ HSV inoculation was similar, although slightly decreased compared to the number after TK⁺ HSV inoculation [128]. It remains necessary to investigate other mutants and to perform longitudinal studies, but the presence of LAT expression in ganglion neurons, coupled with the absence of HSV reactivation, suggests that HSV TK expression is important for reactivation of HSV from latently infected ganglion neurons. In addition, Leist et al. [52] reports the presence of similar amounts of HSV DNA in ganglia after TK⁻ HSV inoculation, further supporting the conclusion that HSV TK expression is not important for the establishment or maintenance of ganglionic infection. These hybridization observations are consistent with results of early studies in which only the detection of reactivated HSV was used as an indication of the occurrence of latency [71–74, 78], as well as more recent molecular biological studies [50–52, 119, 128] and TK complementation investigations [91–93]. In future studies, it may be possible to determine, more accurately, the function of HSV TK expression in the a

b

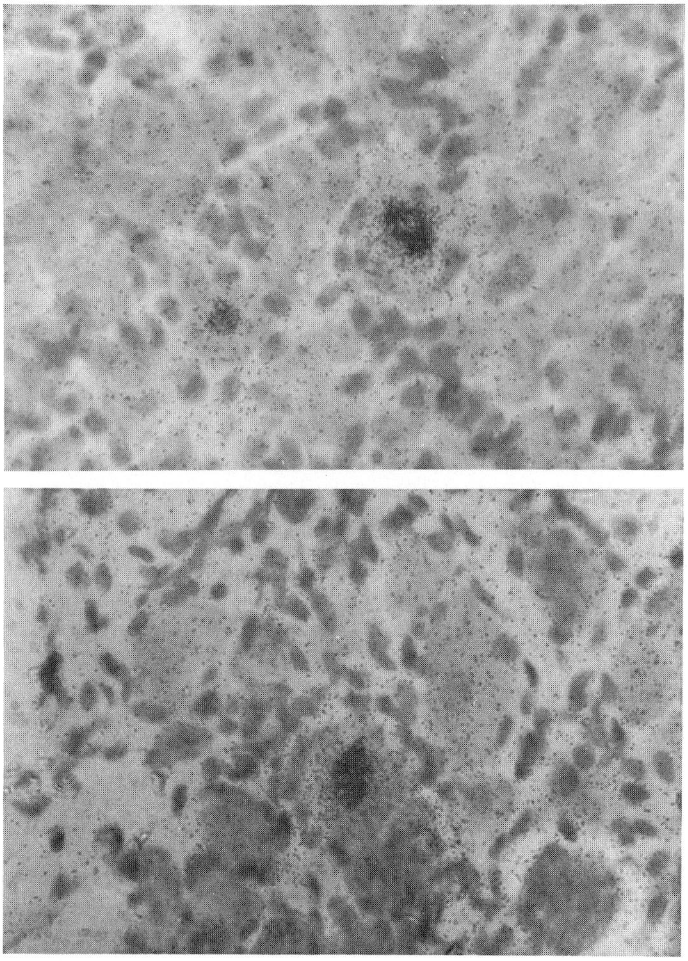

Fig. 2. Detection of HSV-1 LAT in mouse trigeminal ganglion neurons 28 days after corneal inoculation of HSV-1 TK$^-$ mutant. Paraffin ganglion sections were probed with the EC subfragment of the HSV-1 *Bam*HI E fragment **(a)** or with a LAT strand-specific oligonucleotide **(b)**. For the latter, a synthetic 30-mer was used, extending from base 416–445 of the LAT sequence published by Wagner et al. [129]. DNA probes were labeled with [^{35}S], and viruses and hybridization conditions were as described previously [127].

reactivation process by the use of drugs which inhibit the viral TK but not viral replication [130, 131], or by the use of antisense RNA to inhibit HSV TK expression [132, 133].

While recent in situ hybridization studies are very useful in investigating the molecular-biochemical basis of HSV pathogenesis; they have, however, also raised questions about definitions of TK$^-$ HSV latency.

Reactivation Is Part of Latency

In brief, it appears that: (i) TK$^-$ HSV LAT is present in ganglion neurons during latency [51, 52, 128], and by the results of rescue [50, 51] and complementation [91–93] studies, there is evidence that the entire genome may be present; but, (ii) TK$^-$ HSV usually does not reactivate from latency [71–74], leading to the question of; (iii) what is an appropriate designation of a long-term LAT-expressing but reactivation-defective TK^- HSV infection? Although during latency, i.e. during the long-term, quiescent period of infection, there may be little difference between infection by TK^+ and by TK^- HSV. It seems necessary to differentiate between TK^- HSV infection where LAT is expressed but where reactivation is uncommon, from TK^+ HSV infection where reactivation in explants is frequent. Reactivation is the most specific sign of HSV latency and is of considerable importance in pathogenesis, including in humans, and reactivation competence should probably be part of the definition of HSV latency. LAT-expressing, reactivation-defective TK^- HSV infections may be considered 'truly' or 'completely' latent, specifically because reactivation is limited, although we have chosen an alternative nomenclature and have considered such HSV infections as demonstrating incomplete latency [128]. This terminology reflects an emphasis on the importance of HSV reactivation for latency.

It will be of interest to determine the occurrence of other HSV mutants which do not reactivate from ganglia but where viral nucleic acid is present in ganglia and which, therefore, may also establish incomplete latent infections. This has been reported, for example, for an HSV ICP 0 mutant, where mutant virus does not reactivate from latently infected ganglia but where viral DNA was present in ganglion tissue, and virus could be rescued by in vitro superinfection [134]. The emphasis on reactivation may depend in part on methodology, and the use of agents which enhance reactivation in ganglion explants [134, 135] may alter whether a given infection is considered to be latent or incompletely latent. In addition it may be noted that an emphasis on viral reactivation for HSV latency leaves latent infection of the central nervous system (brain and spinal cord) with unclear status; reactivation of latent HSV infection of the central nervous system may occur but is considerably less common than is the reactivation from the peripheral nervous system [123, 136–138].

From the information discussed in this review, it is concluded that HSV TK expression, particularly TK expression of HSV-1, is important for the reactivation of latent HSV infection of sensory ganglion neurons, probably because of limited cellular TK expression and absent replication capacity of these cells. TK mutants of HSV may infect ganglion neurons but are usually reactivation defective, and for this reason have been considered to establish incomplete latent infections. The nomenclature of HSV latency remains to be more clearly defined, and this will likely follow further understanding of the mechanisms of latency.

Acknowledgments

Supported in part by Javits Neuroscience Investigator Award NS 20684 and Training Grant CA 09124. The secretarial assistance of Karen Rank and the editorial assistance of Ann Viozzi are appreciated.

References

1 Kit S, Dubbs DR: Acquisition of thymidine kinase activity by herpes simplex infected mouse fibroblast cells. Biochem Biophys Res Commun 1963;11:55–59.
2 Nohara H, Kaplan AS: Induction of a new enzyme in rabbit kidney cells by pseudorabies virus. Biochem Biophys Res Commun 1963;12: 189–193.
3 Dubbs DR, Kit S: Mutant strains of herpes simplex deficient in thymidine kinase-inducing activity. Virology 1964;22:493–502.

4 Klemperer HG, Haynes GR, Shedden WIH, Watson DH: A virus-specific thymidine kinase in BHK21 cells infected with herpes simplex virus. Virology 1967;31:120–128.
5 Buchan A, Watson DH: The immunological specificity of thymidine kinases in cells infected by viruses of the herpes group. J Gen Virol 1969; 4:461–463.
6 Thouless ME, Skinner GRB: Differences in the properties of thymidine kinase produced by cells infected with type 1 and type 2 herpes virus. J Gen Virol 1971;12:195–197.
7 Ogino T, Rapp F: Differences in thermal stability of deoxythymidine kinase activity in extracts from cell infected with herpes simplex virus type 1 or type 2. Virology 1971;46:953–955.
8 Dobersen MJ, Jerkofsky M, Greer S: Enzymatic basis for the selective inhibition of varicella-zoster virus by 5-halogenated analogues of deoxycytidine. J Virol 1976;20:478–486.
9 Sawyer MH, Inchauspe G, Biron KK, Waters DJ, Straus SE, Ostrove JM: Molecular analysis of the pyrimidine deoxyribonucleoside kinase gene of wild-type and acyclovir-resistant strains of varicella-zoster virus. J Gen Virol 1988;69: 2585–2593.
10 Mori H, Shiraki K, Kato T, Hayakawa Y, Yamanishi K, Takahaski M: Molecular analysis of the thymidine kinase gene of thymidine kinase-deficient mutants of varicella-zoster virus. Intervirology 1988;29:301–310.
11 Roubal J, Klein G: Synthesis of thymidine kinase (TK) in Epstein-Barr virus-superinfected Raji TK-negative cells. Intervirology 1981;15: 43–48.
12 Ooka T, Calender A, de Turenne M, Daillie J: Effect of arabinofuranosylthymine on the replication of Epstein-Barr virus and relationship with a new induced thymidine kinase activity. J Virol 1983;46:187–195.
13 Littler E, Zeuthen J, McBride AA, Sorensen ET, Powell KL, Walsh-Arrand JE, Arrand JR: Identification of an Epstein-Barr virus-coded thymidine kinase. EMBO J 1986;5:1959–1966.
14 Lomniczi B, Kaplan AS, Ben-Porat T: Multiple defects in the genome of pseudorabies virus can affect virulence without detectably affecting replication in cell culture. Virology 1987;161: 181–189.
15 Allen GP, McGowan JJ, Gentry GA, Randall CC: Biochemical transformation of deoxythymidine kinase-deficient mouse cells with UV-irradiated equine herpesvirus type 1. J Virol 1978; 28:361–367.
16 McGowan JJ, Allen GP, Barnett JM, Gentry GA: Deoxythymidine kinase metabolism in equine herpesvirus type 3 infected horse embryo dermal fibroblasts. Virology 1980;101:516–519.
17 Weinmaster GA, Misra V, McGuire R, Babiuk LA, DeClercq E: Bovid herpesvirus type-1 (infectious bovine rhinotracheitis virus) - induced thymidine kinase. Virology 1982;118:191–201.
18 Mittal SK, Field HJ: Analysis of the bovine herpesvirus type 1 thymidine kinase (TK) gene from wild-type virus and TK-deficient mutants. J Gen Virol 1989;70:901–918.
19 Scott SD, Ross NLJ, Binns MM: Nucleotide and predicted amino sequences of the Marek's disease virus and turkey herpesvirus thymidine kinase genes: Comparison with thymidine kinase genes of other herpesviruses. J Gen Virol 1989; 70:3055–3065.
20 Kit S, Kit M, Ichimura H, Crandell R, McConnell S: Induction of thymidine kinase activity by viruses with group B DNA genomes: bovine cytomegalovirus (bovine herpesvirus 4). Virus Res 1986;4:197–212.
21 Kit S, Jorgensen GN, Leung W-C, Trkula D, Dubbs DR: Thymidine kinases induced by avian and human herpesviruses. Intervirology 1973/1974;2:299–311.
22 Martin SL, Aparisio DI, Bandyopadhyay PK: Genetic and biochemical characterization of the thymidine kinase gene from herpesvirus of turkeys. J Virol 1989;63:2847–2852.
23 Sheppard M, May JT: Location and characterization of the bovine herpesvirus type 2 thymidine kinase. J Gen Virol 1989;70:3067–3071.
24 Nunberg JH, Wright DK, Cole GE, Petrovskis EA, Post LE, Compton T, Gilbert JH: Identification of the thymidine kinase gene of feline herpesvirus: Use of degenerate oligonucleotides in the polymerase chain reaction to isolate herpesvirus gene homologs. J Virol 1989;63: 3240–3249.
25 Otsuka H, Kit S: Nucleotide sequence of the marmoset herpesvirus thymidine kinase gene and predicted amino acid sequence of thymidine kinase polypeptide. Virology 1984;135:316–330.
26 Honess RW, O'Hare PO, Young D: Comparison

of thymidine kinase activities induced in cells productively infected with herpesvirus saimiri and herpes simplex virus. J Gen Virol 1982;58: 237–249.
27 Buller RML, Smith GL, Cremer K, Notkins AL, Moss B: Decreased virulence of recombinant vaccinia virus expression vectors is associated with a thymidine kinase-negative phenotype. Nature 1985;317:813–815.
28 Binns MM, Tomley FM, Campbell J, Boursnell MEG: Comparison of a conserved region in fowlpox virus and vaccinia virus genomes and the translocation of the fowlpox virus thymidine kinase gene. J Gen Virol 1988;69:1275–1283.
29 Munyon W, Kraiselburd E, Davis D, Mann J: Transfer of thymidine kinase to thymidine kinaseless L cells by infection with ultraviolet-irradiated herpes simplex virus. J Virol 1971;7: 813–820.
30 Bacchetti S, Graham FL: Transfer of the gene for thymidine kinase to thymidine kinase-deficient human cells by purified herpes simplex viral DNA. Proc Natl Acad Sci USA 1977;74: 1590–1594.
31 Maitland NJ, McDougall JK: Biochemical transformation of mouse cells by fragments of herpes simplex virus DNA. Cell 1977;11: 233–241.
32 Pellicer A, Wigler M, Axel R, Silverstein S: The transfer and stable integration of the HSV thymidine kinase gene into mouse cells. Cell 1978; 14:133–141.
33 Wigler M, Silverstein S, Lee L-S, Pellicer A, Cheng Y-C, Axel R: Transfer of purified herpes virus thymidine kinase gene to cultured mouse cells. Cell 1977;11:223–232.
34 Halliburton IW, Morse LS, Roizman B, Quinn KE: Mapping of the thymidine kinase genes of type 1 and type 2 herpes simplex viruses using intertypic recombinants. J Gen Virol 1980;49: 235–253.
35 McDougall JK, Masse TH, Galloway DA: Location and cloning of the herpes simplex virus type 2 thymidine kinase gene. J Virol 1980;33: 1221–1224.
36 Reyes GR, Jeang K-T, Hayward GS: Transfection with the isolated herpes simplex virus thymidine kinase genes. I. Minimal size of the active fragments from HSV-1 and HSV-2. J Gen Virol 1982;62:191–206.
37 McKnight SL: The nucleotide sequence and transcript map of the herpes simplex virus thymidine kinase gene. Nucl Acids Res 1980;8: 5949–5964.
38 Wagner MJ, Sharp JA, Summers WC: Nucleotide sequence of the thymidine kinase gene of herpes simplex virus type 1. Proc Natl Acad Sci USA 1981;78:1441–1445.
39 Swain MA, Galloway DA: Nucleotide sequence of the herpes simplex virus type 2 thymidine kinase gene. J Virol 1983;46:1045–1050.
40 Gompels U, Minson A: The properties and sequence of glycoprotein H of herpes simplex virus type 1. Virology 1986;153:230–247.
41 Darby G, Larder BA, Inglis MM: Evidence that the 'active centre' of the herpes simplex virus thymidine kinase involves an interaction between three distinct regions of the polypeptide. J Gen Virol 1986;67:753–758.
42 Graessmann A, Graessmann M: DNA methylation, chromatin structure and regulation of herpes simplex virus tk gene expression. Gene 1988;74:135–137.
43 de Jong JT, Aker J, den Dulk H, van de Putte P, Giphart-Gassler M: Cytosine methylation in the EcoR 1 site of active and inactive herpesvirus thymidine kinase promoters. Biochem Biophys Acta 1989;1008:62–70.
44 Cremer KJ, Bodemer M, Summers WP, Summers WC, Gesteland RF: In vitro suppression of UAG and UGA mutants in the thymidine kinase gene of herpes simplex virus. Proc Natl Acad Sci USA 1979;76:430–434.
45 McKnight SL, Gavis ER: Expression of the herpes thymidine kinase gene in Xenopus laevis oocytes: An assay for the study of deletion mutants constructed in vitro. Nucl Acids Res 1980; 8:5931–5948.
46 Shih M-F, Arsenakis M, Tiollais P, Roizman B: Expression of hepatitis B virus S gene by herpes simplex virus type 1 vectors carrying α and β regulated gene chimeras. Proc Natl Acad Sci USA 1984;81:5867–5870.
47 ElKareh A, Murphy AJM, Fichter T, Efstratiadis A: 'Transactivation' control signals in the promoter of the herpesvirus thymidine kinase gene. Proc Natl Acad Sci USA 1985;82:1002–1006.
48 Smiley JR: Construction in vitro and rescue of a thymidine kinase-deficient deletion mutation

of herpes simplex virus. Nature 1980;285: 333–335.

49 Post LE, Mackem S, Roizman B: Regulation of α genes of herpes simplex virus: Expression of chimeric genes produced by fusion of thymidine kinase with α gene promotors. Cell 1981;24: 555–565.

50 Efstathiou S, Kemp S, Darby G, Minson AC: The role of herpes simplex virus type 1 thymidine kinase in pathogenesis. J Gen Virol 1989;70: 869–879.

51 Coen DM, Kosz-Vnenchak M, Jacobson JG, Leib DA, Bogard CL, Schaffer PA, Tyler KL, Knipe DM: Thymidine kinase-negative herpes simplex virus mutants establish latency in mouse trigeminal ganglia but do not reactivate. Proc Natl Acad Sci USA 1989;86:4736–4740.

52 Leist TP, Sandri-Goldin RM, Stevens JG: Latent infections in spinal ganglia with thymidine kinase-deficient herpes simplex virus. J Virol 1989;63:4976–4978.

53 Heyman RA, Borrelli E, Lesley J, Anderson D, Richman DD, Baird SM, Hyman R, Evans RM: Thymidine kinase obliteration: Creation of transgenic mice with controlled immune deficiency. Proc Natl Acad Sci USA 1989;86: 2698–2702.

54 Borrelli E, Heyman RA, Arias C, Sawchenko PE, Evans RM: Transgenic mice with inducible dwarfism. Nature 1989;339:538–541.

55 Honess RW, Watson DN: Herpes simplex virus-specific polypeptides studied by polyacrylamide gel electrophoresis of immune precipitates. J Gen Virol 1974;22:171–185.

56 Summers WP, Wagner M, Summers WC: Possible peptide chain termination mutants in thymidine kinase gene of a mammalian virus, herpes simplex virus. Proc Natl Acad Sci USA 1975; 72:4081–4084.

57 Cheng Y-C, Ostrander M: Deoxythymidine kinase induced in HeLa TK⁻ cells by herpes simplex virus type I and type II. J Biol Chem 1976;251:2605–2610.

58 Sanderson MR, Freemont PS, Murthy HMK, Krane JF, Summers WC, Steitz TA: Purification and crystallization of thymidine kinase from herpes simplex virus type 1. J Mol Biol 1988; 202:917–919.

59 Chen MS, Prusoff WH: Association of thymidine kinase activity with pyrimidine deoxyribonucleoside kinase induced by herpes simplex virus. J Biol Chem 1978;253:1325–1327.

60 Chen MS, Summers WP, Walker J, Summers WC, Prusoff WH: Characterization of pyrimidine deoxyribonucleoside kinase (thymidine kinase) and thymidine kinase as a multifunctional enzyme in cells transformed by herpes simplex virus type 1 and in cells infected with mutant strains of herpes simplex virus. J Virol 1979; 30:942–945.

61 Cooper GM: Phosphorylation of 5-bromodeoxycytidine in cells infected with herpes simplex virus. Proc Natl Acad Sci USA 1973;70: 3788–3792.

62 Jamieson AT, Gentry GA, Subak-Sharpe JH: Induction of both thymidine and deoxycytidine kinase activity by herpes viruses. J Gen Virol 1974;24:465–480.

63 Cheng Y-C: A rational approach to the development of antiviral chemotherapy: alternative substrates of herpes simplex virus type 1 (HSV-1) and type 2 (HSV-2) thymidine kinase (TK). Ann NY Acad Sci 1977;284:594–598.

64 Coen DM, Fleming HE Jr, Leslie LK, Retondo MJ: Sensitivity of arabinosyladenine-resistant mutants of herpes simplex virus to other antiviral drugs and mapping of drug hypersensitivity mutations to the DNA polymerase locus. J Virol 1985;53:477–488.

65 Elion GB, Furman PA, Fyfe JA, deMiranda P, Beauchamp L, Schaeffer HJ: Selectivity of action of an antiherpetic agent 9-(2-hydroxyethoxymethyl)guanine. Proc Natl Acad Sci USA 1977;74:5716–5720.

66 Fyfe JA, Keller PM, Furman PA, Miller RL, Elion GB: Thymidine kinase from herpes simplex virus phosphorylates the new antiviral compound 9-(2-hydroxyethoxymethyl)guanine. J Biol Chem 1978;253:8721–8727.

67 Derse D, Cheng Y-C, Furman PA, St Clair MH, Elion GB: Inhibition of purified human and herpes simplex virus-induced DNA polymerases by 9-(2-hydroxyethoxymethyl)guanine triphosphate. Effects on primer-template function. J Biol Chem 1981;256:11447–11451.

68 Kit S: Thymidine kinase. Microbiol Sci 1985; 2:369–375.

69 Marcialis MA, LaColla P, Schivo ML, Flore O, Firinu A, Loddo B: Low virulence and immunogenicity in mice and in rabbits of variants of

herpes simplex virus resistant to 5-iodo-2-deoxyuridine. Experientia 1975;31:502–503.
70 Field HJ, Wildy P: The pathogenicity of thymidine kinase-deficient mutants of herpes simplex virus in mice. J Hyg 1978;81:267–277.
71 Tenser RB, Miller RL, Rapp F: Trigeminal ganglion infection by thymidine kinase-negative mutants of herpes simplex virus. Science 1979; 205:915–917.
72 Tenser RB, Dunstan ME: Herpes simplex virus thymidine kinase expression in infection of the trigeminal ganglion. Virology 1979;99:417–422.
73 Field HJ, Darby G: Pathogenicity in mice of strains of herpes simplex virus which are resistant to acyclovir in vitro and in vivo. Antimicrob Agents Chemother 1980;17:209–216.
74 Klein RJ, DeStefano E, Brady E, Friedman-Kien AE: Experimental skin infection with an acyclovir resistant herpes simplex virus mutant: Response to antiviral treatment and protection against reinfection. Arch Virol 1980;65: 237–246.
75 Darby G, Field HJ, Salisbury SA: Altered substrate specificity of herpes simplex virus thymidine kinase confers acyclovir-resistance. Nature 1981;289:81–83.
76 Tenser RB: Intracerebral inoculation of newborn and adult mice with thymidine kinase-deficient mutants of herpes simplex virus type 1. J Infect Dis 1983;147:956.
77 Gordon YJ, Gilden DM, Becker Y: HSV-1 thymidine kinase promotes virulence and latency in the mouse. Invest Ophthalmol Vis Sci 1983; 24:599–602.
78 Tenser RB, Jones JC, Ressel SJ: Acute and latent infection by thymidine kinase mutants of herpes simplex virus type 2. J Infect Dis 1985;151: 548–550.
79 Halliburton IW, Honess RW, Killington RA: Virulence is not conserved in recombinants between herpes simplex virus types 1 and 2. J Gen Virol 1987;68:1435–1440.
80 Sakuma S, Yamamoto M, Kumano Y, Mori R: An acyclovir-resistant strain of herpes simplex virus type 2 which is highly virulent for mice. Arch Virol 1988;101:169–182.
81 Izumi KM, Stevens JG: Two thymidine kinase deficient herpes simplex viruses exhibit unexpected virulence properties. Microbiol Pathogen 1988;4:145–153.
82 Tenser RB, Ressel SJ, Fralish FA, Jones JC: The role of pseudorabies virus thymidine kinase expression in trigeminal ganglion infection. J Gen Virol 1983;64:1369–1373.
83 Kit S, Kit M, Pirtle EC: Attenuated properties of thymidine kinase-negative deletion mutant of pseudorabies virus. Am J Vet Res 1985;46: 1359–1367.
84 Stevens JG, Cook ML: Latent herpes simplex virus in spinal ganglia of mice. Science 1971; 173:843–845.
85 Stevens JG, Nesburn AB, Cook ML: Latent herpes simplex virus from trigeminal ganglia of rabbits with recurrent eye infection. Nature New Biol 1972;235:216–217.
86 Dundarov S, Dundarova D, Todorov S, Kavaklova L, Falke D: Induction capacity and influence of dThdMP on thymidine kinase activity of type 1 and 2 strains of herpes simplex virus. Arch Virol 1978;56:243–249.
87 Tenser RB, Ressel S, Dunstan ME: Herpes simplex virus thymidine kinase expression in trigeminal ganglion infection: correlation of enzyme activity with ganglion virus titer and evidence of in vivo complementation. Virology 1981;112:328–341.
88 Tenser Rb, Edris WA: Thymidine kinase (TK) activity in herpes simplex virus type 1 recombinants that carry insertions affecting regulation of the TK gene. Virology 1986;155:257–261.
89 Martin JL, Ellis MN, Keller PM, Biron KK, Lehrman SN, Barry DW, Furman PA: Plaque autoradiography assay for the detection and quantitation of thymidine kinase-deficient and thymidine kinase – altered mutants of herpes simplex virus in clinical isolates. Antimicrob Agents Chemother 1985;28:181–187.
90 Coen DM, Irmiere AF, Jacobson JG, Kerns KM: Low levels of herpes simplex virus thymidine-thymidylate kinase are not limiting for sensitivity to certain antiviral drugs or for latency in a mouse model. Virology 1989;168:221–231.
91 Field HJ, Lay E: Characterization of latent infections in mice inoculated with herpes simplex virus which is clinically resistant to acyclovir. Antiviral Res 1984;4:43–52.
92 Tenser RB, Edris WA: Trigeminal ganglion infection by thymidine kinase-negative mutants of herpes simplex virus after in vivo complementation. J Virol 1987;61:2171–2174.

93 Ellis MN, Waters R, Hill EL, Lobe DC, Selleseth DW, Barry DW: Orofacial infection of athymic mice with defined mixtures of acyclovir-susceptible and acyclovir-resistant herpes simplex virus type 1. Antimicrob Agents Chemother 1989; 33:304–310.
94 Jamieson AT, Subak-Sharpe JH: Interallelic complementation of mutants of herpes simplex virus deficient in deoxypyrimidine kinase activity. Virology 1978;85:109–117.
95 Gronowitz JS, Kallander CFR: Optimized assay for thymidine kinase and its application to the detection of antibodies against herpes simplex virus type 1- and 2-induced thymidine kinase. Infect Immun 1980;29:425–434.
96 Veerisetty V, Gentry GA: Alterations in substrate specificity and physicochemical properties of deoxythymidine kinase of a drug-resistant herpes simplex virus type 1 mutant. J Virol 1983;46:901–908.
97 Miller RL, Iltis JP, Rapp F: Differential effect of arabinofuranosylthymine on the replication of human herpesviruses. J Virol 1977;23:679–684.
98 Cheng Y-C, Schinazi RF, Dutschman GE, Tan RS, Grill SP: Virus-induced thymidine kinases as markers for typing herpes simplex viruses and for drug sensitivity assays. J Virol Methods 1982;5:209–217.
99 Summers WC, Summers WP: [^{125}I] deoxycytidine used in a rapid, sensitive, and specific assay for herpes simplex virus type 1 thymidine kinase. J Virol 1977;24:314–318.
100 Tenser RB, Jones JC, Ressel SJ, Fralish FA: Thymidine plaque autoradiography of thymidine kinase-positive and thymidine kinase-negative herpesviruses. J Clin Microbiol 1983;17: 122–127.
101 Fang Z-Y, Tenser RB, Rapp F: Hepatic infection by thymidine kinase-positive and thymidine kinase-negative herpes simplex virus after partial hepatectomy. Infect Immun 1983;42: 402–408.
102 Watson K, Stevens JG, Cook ML, Subak-Sharpe JH: Latency competence of thirteen HSV-1 temperature-sensitive mutants. J Gen Virol 1980; 49:149–159.
103 McLennan JL, Darby G: Herpes simplex virus latency: the cellular location of virus in dorsal root ganglia and the fate of the infected cell following virus activation. J Gen Virol 1980; 51:233–243.
104 Steiner I, Spivack JG, Deshmane SL, Ace CI, Preston CM, Fraser NW: A herpes simplex virus type 1 mutant containing a nontransinducing Vmw65 protein establishes latent infection in vivo in the absence of viral replication and reactivates efficiently from explanted trigeminal ganglia. J Virol 1990;64:1630–1638.
105 Price RW, Khan A: Resistance of peripheral autonomic neurons to in vivo productive infection by herpes simplex virus mutants deficient in thymidine kinase activity. Infect Immun 1981;34:571–580.
106 Gordon YJ, Rao H, Arullo-Cruz T: Immunosuppression promotes ocular virus replication and CNS neurovirulence following corneal inoculation with an avirulent herpes simplex type 1 thymidine kinase negative mutant. Curr Eye Res 1984;3:651–657.
107 Stanberry LR, Kit S, Myers MG: Thymidine-kinase deficient herpes simplex virus type 2 genital infection in guinea pigs. J Virol 1985;55: 322–328.
108 Sears AE, Meignier B, Roizman B: Establishment of latency in mice by herpes simplex virus 1 recombinants that carry insertions affecting regulation of the thymidine kinase gene. J Virol 1985;55:410–416.
109 Meignier B, Longnecker R, Roizman B: In vivo behavior of genetically engineered herpes simplex viruses R7017 and R7020: construction and evaluation in rodents. J Infect Dis 1988;158: 602–614.
110 Erlich KS, Mills J, Chatis P, Mertz GJ, Busch DF, Follansbee SE, Grant RM, Crumpacker CS: Acyclovir-resistant herpes simplex virus infection in patients with the acquired immunodeficiency disease syndrome. N Engl J Med 1989;320:293–296.
111 Burns WH, Santos GW, Saral R, Laskin OL, Lietman PS, McLaren C, Barry DW: Isolation and characterization of resistant herpes simplex virus after acyclovir therapy. Lancet 1982;i: 421–423.
112 Westheim AI, Tenser RB, Marks JG Jr: Acyclovir resistance in a patient with chronic mucocutaneous herpes simplex infection. J Am Acad Dermatol 1987;17:875–880.

113 Larder BA, Derse D, Cheng Y-C, Darby G: Properties of purified enzymes induced by pathogenic drug-resistant mutants of herpes simplex virus. J Biol Chem 1983;258:2027–2033.
114 Field H, McMillan A, Darby G: The sensitivity of acyclovir-resistant mutants of herpes simplex virus to other antiviral drugs. J Infect Dis 1981;143:281–285.
115 Coen DM, Schaffer PA: Two distinct loci confer resistance to acycloguanosine in herpes simplex virus type 1. Proc Natl Acad Sci USA 1980; 77:2265–2269.
116 Crumpacker CS, Kowalsky PN, Oliver SA, Schnipper LE, Field AK: Resistance of herpes simplex virus to a 9-{[2-hydroxyl-1-(hydroxymethyl)ethoxy]methyl} guanine: Physical mapping of drug synergism within the viral DNA polymerase locus. Proc Natl Acad Sci USA 1984; 81:1556–1560.
117 Larder BA, Cheng Y-C, Darby G: Characterization of abnormal thymidine kinases induced by drug-resistant strains of herpes simplex virus type 1. J Gen Virol 1983;64:523–532.
118 Darby G, Churcher MJ, Larder BA: Cooperative effects between two acyclovir resistance loci in herpes simplex virus. J Virol 1984;50:838–846.
119 Ho DY, Mocarski ES: β-Galactosidase as a marker in the peripheral and neural tissues of the herpes simplex virus-infected mouse. Virology 1988;167:279–283.
120 Galloway DA, Fenoglio C, Shevchuk M, McDougall JK: Detection of herpes simplex RNA in human sensory ganglia. Virology 1979;95:265–268.
121 Tenser RB, Dawson M, Ressel SJ, Dunstan ME: Detection of herpes simplex virus mRNA in latently infected trigeminal ganglion neurons by in situ hybridization. Ann Neurol 1982;11: 285–291.
122 Stevens JG, Wagner EK, Devi-Rao GB, Cook ML, Feldman LT: RNA complementary to a herpesvirus alpha gene mRNA is prominent in latently infected neurons. Science 1987;235: 1056–1059.
123 Deatly AM, Spivack JG, Lavi E, O'Boyle II DR, Fraser NW: Latent herpes simplex virus type 1 transcripts in peripheral and central nervous system tissues of mice map to similar regions of the viral genome. J Virol 1988;62:749–756.
124 Wechsler SL, Nesburn AB, Watson R, Slanina SM, Ghiasi H: Fine mapping of the latency-related gene of herpes simplex virus type 1: Alternative splicing produces distinct latency-related RNAs containing open reading frames. J Virol 1988;62:4051–4058.
125 Gordon YJ, Johnson B, Romanowski E, Araullo-Cruz T: RNA complementary to herpes simplex virus type 1 ICPO gene demonstrated in neurons of human trigeminal ganglia. J Virol 1988;62: 1832–1835.
126 Krause PR, Croen KD, Straus SE, Ostrove JM: Detection and preliminary characterization of herpes simplex virus type 1 transcripts in latently infected human trigeminal ganglia. J Virol 1988;62:4819–4823.
127 Leib DA, Bogard CL, Kosz-Vnenchak M, Hicks KA, Coen DM, Knipe DM, Schaffer PA: A deletion mutant of the latency-associated transcript of herpes simplex virus type 1 reactivates from the latent state with reduced frequency. J Virol 1989;63:2893–2900.
128 Tenser RB, Hay KA, Edris WA: Latency-associated transcript but not reactivatable virus is present in sensory ganglion neurons after inoculation of thymidine kinase-negative mutants of herpes simplex virus type 1. J Virol 1989;63: 2861–2865.
129 Wagner EK, Flanagan WM, Devi-Rao G, Zhang Y-F, Hill JM, Anderson KP, Stevens JG: The herpes simplex virus latency-associated transcript is spliced during the latent phase of infection. J Virol 1988;62:4577–4585.
130 Nutter LM; Grill SP, Dutschman GE, Sharma RA, Bobek M, Cheng Y-C: Demonstration of viral thymidine kinase inhibitor and its effect on deoxynucleotide metabolism in cells infected with herpes simplex virus. Antimicrob Agents Chemother 1987;31:368–374.
131 Martin JA, Duncan IB, Hall MJ, Wong-Kai-In P, Lambert RW, Thomas GJ: New potent and selective inhibitors of herpes simplex virus thymidine kinase. Nucleosides Nucleotides 1989;8: 753–764.
132 Izant JG, Weintraub H: Inhibition of thymidine kinase gene expression by anti-sense RNA: A molecular approach to genetic analysis. Cell 1984;36:1007–1015.
133 Kim SK, Wold BJ: Stable reduction of thymidine kinase activity in cells expressing high levels of anti-sense RNA. Cell 1985;42:129–138.

134 Leib DA, Coen DM, Bogard CL, Hicks KA, Yager DR, Knipe DM, Tyler KL, Schaffer PA: Immediate-early regulatory gene mutants define different stages in the establishment and reactivation of herpes simplex virus latency. J Virol 1989;63:759–768.
135 Whitby AJ, Blyth WA, Hill TJ: The effect of DNA hypomethylating agents on the reactivation of herpes simplex virus from latently infected mouse ganglia in vitro. Arch Virol 1987;97:137–144.
136 Cook ML, Stevens JG: Latent herpetic infections following experimental viraemia. J Gen Virol 1976;31:75–80.
137 Tenser RB, Hsiung GD: Pathogenesis of latent herpes simplex virus infection of the trigeminal ganglion in guinea pigs: effects of age, passive immunization and hydrocortisone. Infect Immun 1977;16:69–74.
138 Stroop WG, Rock DL, Fraser NW: Localization of herpes simplex virus in the trigeminal and olfactory systems of the mouse central nervous system during acute and latent infections by in situ hybridization. Lab Invest 1984;51:27–38.

Note Added in Proof

After the completion of this review, Leib et al. reported a study of compounds which inhibit HSV TK expression but which do not or only slightly inhibit HSV replication [see also 130, 131]. [Antimicrob Agents Chemother 1990;34:1285–1286]. Reactivation of HSV from explants of latently infected ganglia was diminished, by these compounds, and this was considered to indicate an important role for HSV TK expression in the reactivation process.

Intervirology 1991;32:93–100

0300–5526/91/0322–0093$2.75/0

Application of Polymerase Chain Reaction Assays to Studies of Herpes simplex Virus Latency

Edouard M. Cantin, Winand Lange, Harry Openshaw

Department of Neurology, City of Hope National Medical Center, Duarte, Calif., USA

Key Words. Herpes simplex virus type 1 · Polymerase chain reaction · Viral latency · Sensory ganglia

Summary. We have amplified herpes simplex virus type 1 (HSV-1) DNA sequences from individual latently infected mouse trigeminal ganglia by polymerase chain reaction (PCR) assays. This report presents two useful modifications in the PCR technique. The first involves the use of two sets of closely spaced, oppositely oriented oligonucleotide primers and two rounds of 20–40 PCR cycles, first with the more widely spaced outer primers and then with the internal nested primers. This method enhanced the sensitivity of PCR detection as shown by assays of HSV-1 sequences in human brain. The second modification was designed to detect selectively HSV-1 sense or anti-sense RNA transcripts when both are present by adding a single primer during an initial reverse-transcriptase-mediated cDNA synthesis reaction. After destruction of the RNA template, standard PCR is initiated by the addition of the second primer and thermus aquaticus DNA polymerase (Taq). We show here applications of both of these modifications to amplify HSV-1 sequences from nervous system tissue.

The characteristic outcome of infection with herpes simplex virus type 1 (HSV-1) is a latent infection which endures for the life of the host. The latent viral genomes, harbored in peripheral sensory ganglia, can reactivate resulting frequently in recurrent mucocutaneous lesions at or in close proximity to the original site of infection. Relatively little is known of the molecular mechanisms underlying the establishment, maintenance and reactivation of latency. Most studies on the molecular basis of latency have used ganglia taken from experimental animals or from man at postmortem examination, and a major impediment has been the low representation of viral sequences making detection of viral DNA and RNA difficult.

Address inquiries to: Dr. Edouard M. Cantin, Department of Neurology, City of Hope National Medical Center, 1500 East Duarte Road, Duarte, CA 91010–0269 (USA)

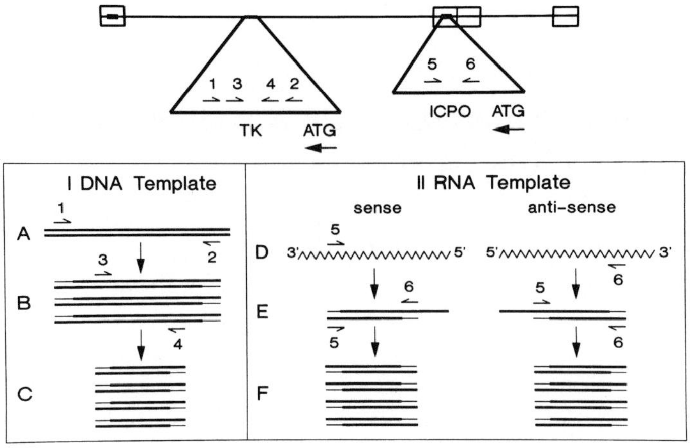

Fig. 1. Schematic depiction of PCR modifications. **A** DNA template. **B** PCR amplification of a 499-bp TK sequence by primers 1 and 2. **C** further PCR amplification of a 273 sequence by the nested primers 3 and 4. **D** RNA templates (sense and anti-sense) with a single primer in the presence of reverse transcriptase. **E** DNA template after destruction of RNA template and reverse transcriptase and addition of second primer. **F** PCR amplification of a 266-bp ICPO sequence by primers 5 and 6. Primer 5 detects anti-sense transcripts whereas primer 6 detects sense transcripts. The restriction endonuclease recognition sequence for *Bam*H1 or *Hin*dIII has been appended to the 5′-end of primers 5 and 6, respectively. The TK primer and probe sequences are as follows: P1 5′ – AATCGCGAACATCTACACCAC – 3′; P2 5′ – AAAGCTGTCCCCTTACCTCCC – 3′; P3 5′ – CTGCAGATACCGCTCCGTATT – 3′; P4 5′ – CATCTTCGACCGCCATCCCAT – 3′; probe 5′ – GTCAAGCTGCCCATAAGGTAT – 3′. The ICPO primer and probe sequences are as follows: P5 5′ – GGATCCTCACGTGGTTACCCGCGGTCT – 3′; P6 5′ – AAGCTTCCGGGGCCGTCCCCGCGGGCG – 3′; probe: 5′ – CCGGCTGGAGCCGCCGCACCCTGCT – 3′-end.

We have used the very sensitive polymerase chain reactions (PCR) technique to detect HSV-1 DNA and RNA sequences in a variety of tissues obtained from experimental animals and from man. The PCR assay originally described by Saiki et al. [1] to amplify a β-globin genomic sequence uses a pair of convergent oligonucleotide primers to amplify a short segment of DNA, the length of which is defined by the distance between the 5′ ends of the primers. The reaction is initiated by template denaturation facilitating annealing of the primers which are then extended with the heat-stable thermus aquaticus DNA polymerase (Taq). Repeated cycles of denaturation, primer annealing, and extension result in an exponential accumulation of the target sequence. The relationship between the extent of amplification (y), the efficiency of the reaction (x), and the number of cycles (n) is $y = (1 + x)^n$. In this report, we present two modifications of the PCR technique applied to HSV latency: (a) the use of nested primers to increase further the sensitivity of PCR detection, and (b) specific amplification of sequences from sense and antisense HSV-1 transcripts when both are present. These modifications are shown in schematic form in figure 1. Oligonucleotide primers and probes were designed on the basis

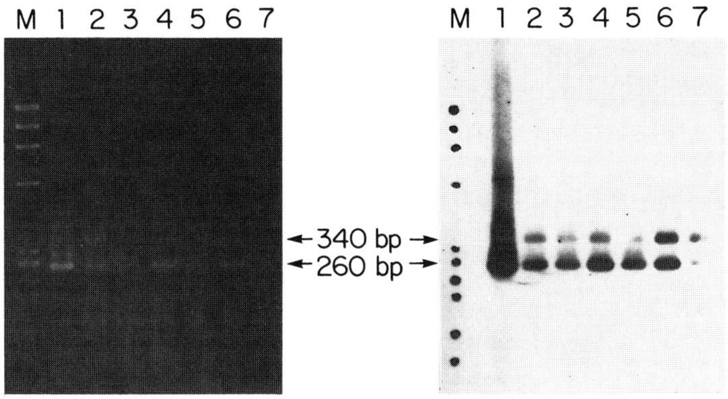

Fig. 2. PCR detection of HSV-1 ICPO sequences in individual latently infected mouse ganglia. Ethidium bromide stained gel (left panel). Southern blot hybridization using mixed ICPO and actin oligonucleotide probes, (right panel). Lanes: M = ΦX174 molecular weight marker; 1 = 100 pg HSV-1 *Bam*-B fragment containing the ICPO gene; 2–7 = DNA extracted from individual latently infected mouse ganglia. HSV-1 ICPO sequence, 260 bp; cellular β-actin sequence, 340 bp. The PCR reaction contained 10 m*M* Tris pH 8.3, 50 m*M* KCl, 1.5 m*M* $MgCl_2$, 0.01% (w/v) gelatin, each dNTP at 200 μ*M* and 20 pmole of each oligonucleotide in a 50-μl reaction. The Mg^{2+} concentration was optimized for each set of primers using the standard cycling program recommended by the thermal cycler manufacturer (Perkin-Elmer-Cetus). Using the optimal Mg^{2+} concentration, other parameters such as primer concentration, annealing temperature, substrate concentration and PCR cycle parameters were optimized for each set of primers. Generally, 30–50 cycles of PCR were done using 0.25–1.0 μg of template in a 50 μl reaction.

of published sequence information for the HSV-1 immediate early ICPO gene [2] and the early thymidine kinase (TK) gene [3].

To detect HSV-1 sequences in latently infected ganglia, we have used 27 bp synthetic oligonucleotide primers 5 and 6 (fig. 1) to amplify a sequence from the HSV-1 ICPO gene of 260 bp in length (excluding bases added for restriction endonuclease recognition sequences). In the example shown in figure 2, DNA was extracted from 6 individual mouse (Balb/c) trigeminal ganglia 2–4 months after inoculation by the corneal route with the F strain of HSV-1. One-fifth of the recovered DNA, estimated to range from 1 to 4 μg, was used as template for 50 cycles of PCR; and one-tenth of each reaction was electrophoresed in a 1.8% agarose gel which was stained with ethidium bromide (fig. 2, left). The DNA was then transferred from the gel to a nylon membrane using an alkaline blotting technique and the membrane hybridized with a ^{32}P-labeled synthetic oligonucleotide probe corresponding to a sequence internal to primers 5 and 6 (fig. 2, right). The 260-bp fragment in lanes 2-7 is the amplified HSV-1 ICPO gene sequence. The reduced signal intensity in lanes 5 and 7 is due in part to a blotting artifact and to the fact that different amounts of DNA were used as template for the PCR. The 340-bp band is a sequence of the cellular β-actin gene which was simultaneously amplified in each reaction by β-actin primers and identified by Southern blot analysis with an internal β-actin probe as a control for the amplification

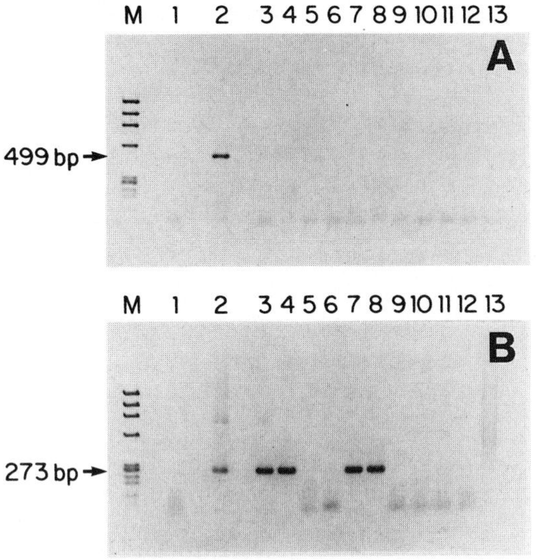

Fig. 3. PCR amplification of HSV-1 TK sequence in DNA extracted from formalin-fixed human brain. **A** Amplification with outer primers 1 and 2 (fig. 1). **B** Additional amplification with nested primers 3 and 4. Lanes: M = ΦX174 molecular weight markers; 1 = primers reacted without DNA template; 2 = pHSV 106 plasmid; 3–12 = brain samples.

competence of the DNA preparation. In all PCR assays a sample lacking DNA/RNA template is included as a contamination control. This sample, as well as a sample containing normal mouse ganglion DNA was negative in the PCR assay.

HSV-1 DNA has been detected in ganglia using various molecular hybridization techniques [4–6]. The enhanced sensitivity of PCR may prove most useful in detecting HSV-1 in extraneural sites not commonly recognized as harboring latent genomes or in nervous system tissue in which there is such a low level of infection that consistent identification of HSV-1 may be achieved only by PCR. For example, explants of ocular tissue occasionally yield HSV-1, and there has been speculation that HSV-1 latency may occur in retinal cells or in the cornea [7–9]. By PCR assays with both the ICPO and TK primers, we have consistently detected HSV-1 DNA in the anterior eye segment (including the cornea) of latently infected mice and occasionally also in the posterior eye segment (including the retina) [10]. Corneal tissue obtained from a limited number of patients undergoing keratoplasty also revealed HSV-1 DNA sequences [Cantin et al., unpubl. results]. Amplification of two different HSV genes facilitates recognition of false positives due mainly to contamination by carryover of PCR reaction products. Our failure to detect HSV-1 RNA transcripts by PCR in the eye of infected littermates argues for bona fide HSV-1 latency rather than a low-level productive HSV-1 infection in the eye. It remains to be determined if such peripheral latency has biological significance, especially in terms of HSV-1 reactivation.

In assays of certain human tissues, we have enhanced the sensitivity of PCR detection by the use of nested primers. The technique using two sets of HSV-1 TK primers is illustrated in figure 1, I and an example is given in figure 3. DNA was extracted from 5-μm sections of formalin-fixed paraffin-embedded brain blocks from patients with AIDS and control non-AIDS brains. Primers 1 and 2 were used initially for 40 cycles of PCR with anticipated amplification of a 499 bp HSV-1 sequence. This fragment can be clearly seen in only lane 2, figure 3A, the pHSV 106 plasmid containing the HSV-1 TK gene, but not in lanes 3–13, containing the PCR reaction products from the brain samples. Southern blot hybridization using a probe internal to primers 1 and 2 was also negative in lanes 3–13 (not shown). When a 1-μl aliquot of a 1:100 dilution of the primary

PCR reaction was re-amplified for an additional 40 cycles with primers 1 and 2, the 499 bp HSV-1 band was present again only in lane 2 (the pHSV 106 plasmid); the brain samples were negative even though there was extensive amplification of cellular sequences as evident as a smear in the ethidium bromide stained gel (not shown). However, when the same dilution of the primary PCR reaction was re-amplified for an additional 40 cycles with the nested TK primers 3 and 4, the anticipated 273-bp fragment was readily detected in 4 of the 11 brain samples in the ethidium bromide stained gel (fig. 3B), and the specificity of this amplification was confirmed by Southern blot hybridization (not shown). This detection in formalin-fixed brain shows that the PCR technique can be successfully carried out with very small amounts of partially degraded DNA samples.

The use of nested primers improves the sensitivity of detection when sequences are present in very low abundance since the increased representation of viral sequence in the second PCR, in conjunction with the use of new primers, minimizes the interfering, nonspecific amplification of cellular sequences. Moreover, nested primers are helpful in the recognition of carryover contamination. This is because the major source of contamination is usually the short product amplified by the nested primers (the 273-bp fragment in fig. 3B), and this short product is not a substrate for the more widely spaced outer set of primers which amplify a larger fragment (499 bp, fig. 3A). A suspected contamination is confirmed if a single PCR assay on the original sample results in a positive signal with the nested primers but not the outer flanking primers.

With the nested primers we have detected HSV-1 TK sequences in both AIDS and non-AIDS cases (fig. 3), none of which had a clinical history of HSV-1 brain infection. Again, the biological significance is uncertain, HSV-1 DNA has previously been detected by liquid-phase hybridization in the brains of latently infected animals after corneal HSV-1 inoculation [11] and also by Southern blot in the brain of humans who had no signs of HSV-1 infection at death [12]. Unlike ganglia, where explantation readily results in in vitro reactivation, HSV-1 is only rarely isolated from explants of brain tissue [11], although in situ reactivation in the brain has been induced experimentally in animals [13].

Using the nested TK primers and ICPO primers, we have also amplified very low levels of HSV-1 sequences in peripheral blood mononuclear cells of normal subjects and patients who have undergone bone marrow transplantation [Cantin et al., 14th International Herpesvirus Workshop, 1989]. Further work is underway to evaluate this additional potential site of extraneural latency.

The second PCR modification discussed in this report involves the selective detection of sense or anti-sense HSV-1 transcripts when both are present. This is shown schematically in figure 1 II, and an example is given in figure 4. A single PCR primer was initially used together with avian myeloblastosis virus (AMV) reverse transcriptase to prime cDNA synthesis from RNA extracted from uninfected (lanes 1 and 2) and infected (lanes 3 and 4) Vero cells, from latently infected mouse trigeminal ganglia (lanes 5 and 6) and from latently infected mouse brain stem (lanes 7 and 8). HSV-1 DNA encoding the RNA transcripts was amplified as an additional positive control (lane 9). After heating at 95° for 5 min to denature the RNA:DNA hybrid, the RNA template was destroyed by

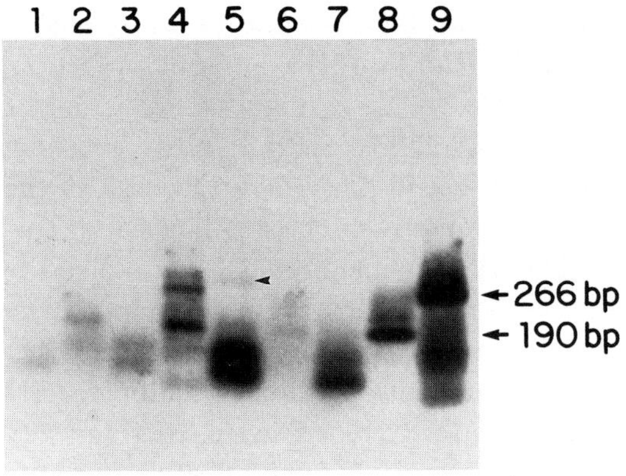

Fig. 4. PCR-selective detection of sense and anti-sense HSV-1 transcripts. Lanes: Odd-numbered 1–7 = anti-sense; even-numbered (2–8) = sense; 1, 2 = uninfected Vero cells; 3, 4 = HSV-1-infected Vero cells; 5, 6 = latently infected mouse ganglia; 7, 8 = latently infected mouse brain stem; 9 = plasmid PBR 112. The RNA-PCR is the same as the DNA-PCR (fig. 2, legend) except that an initial cDNA synthesis step is included to provide the DNA template. Amplification of contaminating DNA is ruled out because different products are obtained depending on which primer is used for cDNA synthesis. Also, omission of the reverse transcriptase step abrogates amplification of the target RNA.

incubation with RNAse for 15 min at 37° and then the second primer and Taq were added for standard PCR cycles of denaturation, primer annealing and primer extension. More recent experiments have shown that the RNAse step is unnecessary; heating suffices to destroy the reverse transcriptase thus precluding amplification of the complementary RNA transcript when the second primer is added. Sense transcripts are assayed when the initial primer is complementary to the non-coding DNA strand (primer 5, even-numbered lanes in fig. 4); and anti-sense transcripts are detected when the initial primer is complementary to the coding DNA strand (primer 6, odd-numbered lanes in fig. 4).

The sense ICPO mRNA transcript (266 bp) was detected only in HSV-infected Vero cells (lane 4) and is indistinguishable in size from the amplified ICPO plasmid product (lane 9). A faint anti-sense HSV-1–specific transcript was detected only in latently infected ganglia (lane 5, arrow) and for unknown reasons appears to be slightly larger (280 bp) than the sense transcript. Unexpectedly, this set of primers also amplified a cellular 'sense' transcript (with respect to the ICPO mRNA) of 190 bp (lanes 2, 4, 6 and 8) which was detected as an ethidium bromide-stained band and which hybridized strongly with the internal oligonucleotide probe even after moderately stringent washing, thus indicating significant sequence similarity to the ICPO gene. This cellular transcript is most likely derived from an intron-containing gene since the ICPO primers failed to amplify a cellular sequence of 190 bp from a DNA template (fig. 2). Very stringent washing of the blot in 3 *M* tetramethylammonium chloride (Me4NCl) completely removed the signal from the 190-bp cellular transcript (not shown). However, Me4NCl washing did not remove the 266-bp sense ICPO transcript (lane 4) or the anti-sense HSV-1-specific transcript (lane 5, arrow). Also preserved were the hybridizations to the low-molecular-weight fragments generated with the anti-sense specific primers (lanes 1, 3, 5 and 7). The origin of these low-molecular-weight hybridizing fragments is unknown, but they could arise from amplification of novel anti-sense transcripts generated by alternate RNA processing or from mispriming events (e.g. Mispriming of the PBR 112 plasmid is seen in fig. 4, lane 9).

There have been several reports in the last 3 years of the detection by Northern blot and in situ hybridization of RNAs in latently infected tissue that are transcribed in the opposite orientation to the ICPO gene and are thus anti-sense transcripts, the 3′-termini of which overlap the 3′-end of ICPO mRNA [14–16]. Initially, these latency-associated transcripts (LATs) were hypothesized to play a role in the establishment and maintenance of latency through an anti-sense mechanism, but later analysis of deletion mutants has suggested their role may be limited to facilitating reactivation [17, 18]. The ICPO primers used in figures 1 and 4 were designed to amplify 3′-terminal sequences of both ICPO and LAT transcripts. Primer 5 is located in the middle of the predicted LAT open reading frame 2 (ORF 2) while primer 6 lies about 75 bp 3′ of ORF 2. It has not been resolved if there are introns in this region encoding the LAT transcript [19–21]. Whether the PCR amplified anti-sense RNA detected in figure 4 (lane 5) is identical to the LAT is currently under investigation. The PCR method described here provides an additional and very sensitive way of identifying LATs and other sense or anti-sense transcripts that my be important in the control of HSV-1 latency.

Acknowledgments

This work was supported by RG 2100 from the National Multiple Sclerosis Society and by EY 08028, EY 05588, and CA 33572 from the National Institutes of Health.

References

1 Saiki RK, Scharf S, Faloona F, et al: Enzymatic amplification of β-globin genomic sequences and restriction site analysis for diagnosis of sickle cell anemia. Science 1985;230:1350–1354.

2 Perry LJ, McGeoch DJ: The DNA sequences of the long repeat region and adjoining parts of the long unique region in the genome of herpes simplex virus type 1. J Gen Virol 1988;69:2831–2846.

3 McGeoch DJ, Dalrymple MA, Davison AJ, et al: The complete DNA sequence of the long unique region in the genome of herpes simplex virus type 1. J Gen Virol 1988;69:1531–1574.

4 Puga A, Rosenthal JD, Openshaw H, et al: Herpes simplex virus DNA and mRNA sequences in acutely and chronically infected trigeminal ganglia of mice. Virol 1978;89:102–111.

5 Galloway DA, Fenoglio CM, McDougall JK: Limited transcription of the herpes simplex virus genome when latent in human sensory ganglia. J Virol 1982;41:686–691.

6 Rock DL, Fraser NW: Latent herpes simplex virus type 1 DNA contains two copies of the virion DNA joint region. J Virol 1985;55:849–852.

7 Openshaw H: Latency of herpes simplex virus in ocular tissue of mice. Infect Immun 1983;39: 960–962.

8 Abghari SZ, Stulting RD: Recovery of herpes simplex virus from ocular tissues of latently infected inbred mice. Invest Opthalmol Vis Sci 1988;29:239–243.

9 O'Brien WJ, Taylor JL: The isolation of herpes simplex virus from rabbit corneas during latency. Invest Opthalmol Vis Sci 1989;30:357–364.

10 Willey DE, Cantin E, Openshaw H: Herpes simplex virus DNA in ocular tissue of latently infected mice. Invest Opthalmol Vis Sci 1989;30(s):215.

11 Cabrera CV, Wohlenberg C, Openshaw H, et al: Herpes simplex virus DNA sequences in the CNS of latently infected mice. Nature 1980; 288: 288–290.

12 Fraser NW, Lawrence WC, Wroblewska Z, et al: Herpes simplex type 1 DNA in human brain tissue. Proc Natl Acad Sci USA 1981;78:6461–6465.

13 Sekizawa T, Openshaw H: Encephalitis resulting from reactivation of latent herpes simplex virus in mice. J Virol 1984;50:263–266.

14 Stevens JG, Wagner EK, Devi-Rao GB, et al: RNA complementary to a herpesvirus alpha gene mRNA is prominent in latently infected neurons. Science 1987;235:1056–1059.

15 Puga A, Notkins AL: Continued expression of a poly(A)^x transcript of herpes simplex virus type 1 in trigeminal ganglia of latently infected ice. J Virol 1987;61:1700–1703.

16 Deatly AM, Spivack JG, Lavi E, et al: RNA from an immediate early region of the type 1 herpes simplex virus genome is present in the trigeminal ganglia of latently infected mice. Proc Natl Acad Sci USA 1987;84:3204–3208.
17 Javier RT, Stevens JG, Dissette VB, et al: A herpes simplex virus transcript abundant in latently infected neurons is dispensable for establishment of the latent state. Virology 1988;166:254–257.
18 Steiner I, Spivack JG, Lirette RP, et al: Herpes simplex virus type 1 latency-associated transcripts are evidently not essential for latent infection. EMBO J 1989;8:505–511.
19 Wechsler SL, Nesburn AB, Watson R, et al: Fine mapping of the latency-related gene of herpes simplex virus type 1: Alternative splicing produces distinct latency-related RNAs containing open reading frames. J Virol 1988;62:4051–4058.
20 Wagner EK, Flanagan WM, Devi-Rao G, et al: The herpes simplex virus latency-associated transcript is spliced during the latent phase of infection. J Virol 1988;62:4577–4585.
21 Wagner EK, Devi-Rao G, Feldman LT, et al: Physical characterization of the herpes simplex virus latency-associated transcript in neurons. J Virol 1988;62:1194–1202.

Intervirology 1991;32:101–115

0300–5526/91/0322–0101$2.75/0

Role of Latency-Associated Transcript in Herpes simplex Virus Infection

Yaw A. Nsiah, Fred Rapp

Department of Microbiology and Immunology, The Pennsylvania State University College of Medicine, Hershey, Pa., USA

Key Words. Latency-associated transcript · Latency · Herpes simplex virus

Summary. Herpes simplex virus (HSV)-specified RNA transcript has been detected by in situ hybridization and by RNA blot analyses in latently infected peripheral nerve ganglia in experimentally infected mice and humans. Physical analysis of the nucleotide sequence, approximately 2,500, indicates possible splicing of the transcript into two overlapping open reading frames (ORF) and the presence of potential promoter elements. The latency-associated transcript, probably, is involved in the maintenance of latent herpes simplex virus infection; however, recent findings indicate that latent-phase transcription is involved in some in vivo reactivation.

Herpes simplex virus (HSV) infection and its subsequent progression to latency in the infected host have been the subject of numerous investigations for many years. The description of HSV infection and its characteristic relationship to the nervous system in the infected host were first suggested by Cushing [1] and Goodpasture [2]. The recurrent and latent nature of herpesvirus infection have been reviewed since that time [3–9]. The epidemiology of HSV infections in man has a number of unusual features. In particular, the recurrent lesions (herpes labialis and herpes genitalis) often reappear at the same peripheral site. These recurrences often are precipitated by stimuli such as fever, excessive exposure to sunlight and stress, and serum antibodies to the virus which remain constant throughout life irrespective of the frequency of recurrent disease. Moreover, during intervals of clinical normality, it was difficult to isolate a virus from peripheral tissues where lesions are prone to occur. Such observations led to the concept that recurrent herpetic diseases arise from endogenous, life-long, 'hidden' or latent infection rather than frequent reinfection with the virus. The natural history of the virus poses a number of fascinating questions:

Address inquiries to: Dr. Y.A. Nsiah, Biology Department, Eastern Conneticut State University, 83 Windham Street, Willimantic, CT 06226-2295 (USA)

(i) What tissues harbor the latent infection? (ii) How is latency established and maintained? (iii) What happens to virus DNA after the acute phase of infection? (iv) What is the nature of the nucleic acid during the latent period – a period marked by possible inactivity within the virus genome? (v) Is the virus genome associated with any host cellular macromolecules? (vi) What is keeping the virus genome from expressing its genetic information? (vii) What controls or signals are involved in the reactivation of latent virus? (viii) What keeps a virus, which shuts off host macromolecular synthesis right after infection, from destroying the host cell? Significant recent advances have been made in approaching these issues by the detection of specific HSV RNA which is expressed during latency. These latency-associated transcripts (LAT) are the primary subject of this report and will be discussed extensively below.

Herpes simplex Virus Pathogenesis

The pathogenesis of infection usually involves virus multiplication at the point of entry. The virus then proceeds to the nerve endings in the area where it localizes within the nuclei of the nerve cell. It is inside the neuronal nuclei where the latent state, probably, is initiated. HSV latency, which has been reviewed comprehensively elsewhere [5, 6], is operationally defined as the stage of the infection where the presence of infectious virus cannot be detected except by explant cocultivation techniques.

The HSV infection which begins with acute or primary infection, involves multiplication of the virus at the site of inoculation. The virus spreads by retrograde axoplasmic transport and colonizes sensory ganglion neurons. During this acute ganglion infection, virus is detected in cell-free homogenates. Following the initial infection, the virus is not eliminated from the host but rather becomes latent. Stevens and Cook [10] were the first to demonstrate that HSV can establish a latent infection in spinal ganglia of mice after inoculation with the virus in the mouse footpad. Infectious virus was detected only by explant cocultivation of the spinal ganglia. Neither viral antigens nor virions were detected by electron microscopy of immunofluorescence in ganglia in vivo. Cook et al. [11], using immunofluorescence, electron microscopy and autoradiography to study latently infected ganglia, showed that viral antigens and nucleic acid appeared first in neurons during reactivation. McLennan and Darby [12] using temperature-sensitive (*ts*) mutants of HSV to produce latent infection in mice cervical ganglia, also showed reactivation of this mutant virus at the nonpermissive temperature, which eliminates the possible spread of the virus, and occurred first in neurons.

The nature of HSV genomic DNA during infection is either episomal, chromatin associated or joining of termini to become concatameric or circular. Recent evidence [13, 14] suggests that during latency, the viral DNA apparently is associated with chromatin-like structures in the nucleus. The episomal nature of latent herpesvirus genome in mice also has been reported [15]. Rock and Fraser [16] using ^{32}P-labeled probes specific for the junction region of the HSV genome, report that the lack of HSV DNA free ends in latently infected mouse brain is due to the joining of the termini. However, Efstathiou et al. [17] reported the finding of junction fragments, confirming earlier by Rock and Fraser [16].

At a later time, the occult latent infection may be reactivated due to nonspecific stimuli. The virus travels back down the axon to the peripheral site and causes a recrudescent lesion. It is believed that a virus-specific thymidine kinase (TK) may play a role in reactivation. Several investigators [18–20] show that TK-negative mutants can establish latency but are unreactivatable or reactivate only to low levels.

HSV latency is a phase where there is no known viral metabolic activity. However, for the last decade, evidence is accumulating which indicates that there is at least a minimum amount of virus-specific gene transcription in HSV latently infected trigeminal ganglia of the peripheral nervous system. Studies which attempt to elucidate the molecular events responsible for the latent state of HSV have shown that there is limited expression of the viral genome during latency. Hybridization analyses demonstrate the presence of an RNA species, known as the LAT or the latency-related (LR) RNA that accumulates to high levels only in the nuclei of latently infected neurons. Recently, this RNA species was found to be dispensable for the establishment of latency [2]. However, no evidence exists to preclude a role for this RNA in the maintenance of the latent state. Expression of HSV LAT during latency will be discussed in detail and is the subject of this review.

Experimental Evidence for LAT

A primary concern of latency is whether or not the virus DNA is actively expressed or transcribed into mRNA in the infected host. One of the first inconclusive documentations for the existence of virus-encoded messenger ribonucleic acid (mRNA) came from Galloway et al. [22]. They demonstrated, by in situ hybridization, the presence of virus-specific mRNA in trigeminal ganglia of humans latently infected with herpes simplex virus type 2 (HSV-2). In subsequent studies, only a limited region (30% of the U_L) of the genome was actively expressed during latency [23]. Even though Galloway and co-workers reported a positive hybridization signal in latent human sensory ganglia, the specificity is doubtful since some of the signal may have been artifactual (based on the location of the signal in the cell). This apparent false positive may have resulted from a lipofuscin effect [24]. During the acute phase of corneal route infection of the mouse, HSV-1 was found in the neurons, the trigeminal ganglia and nerve root, sensory parts of the medulla, and the cerebral cortex. However, in the latent phase, the virus was detected only in the neurons located primarily in the descending nuclei and the mesencephalic nucleus [25]. Additionally, HSV-1-specific RNA was detected in trigeminal ganglia and central nervous system (CNS) neurons in both the acute and the latent phase of infection; DNA was detected only in the acute phase of infection.

The area of the HSV genome, where a positive hybridization signal was detected, is either near or in the region of the genome encoding the virus-specific enzyme TK gene. Tenser et al. [26], using nick-translated probes were able to detect virus-encoded mRNA in latently infected trigeminal ganglionic cells from guinea pigs. The signal detected by in situ hybridization was lost after treating a sample with RNase but not DNase. Futher analysis of the purported virus-encoded mRNA in latently infected mice trigeminal ganglia by Puga and Notkins [27] showed that the transcript being detected originated from DNA sequences in the immediate early (IE) region-IE–1 encoding infected cell polypeptide zero (ICPO). It also was shown that the probes specifically hybridized to the *Bam*HI restriction fragments B and E in the long internal repeat (IR_L) and terminal repeat (TR_L) regions of the HSV genome, which appears to be polyadenylated. It should be noted here that a product of IE-1 is a trans-activating factor that synergistically interacts with Vmw 175 (ICP4), the product of IE gene IE-3 (ICP4) [28]. Consequently, the uncoupling of this interaction may be one of the mechanisms involved in the establishment of latency [28].

In the last 3 years there has been a great deal of experimental evidence to support the presence of LAT or LR RNA. Stevens et al. [29] observed, by in situ hybridization, that ICPO probes hybridized to LAT transcripts, which primarily localized in the nucleus of the infected cells during latency but are found in both nucleus and cytoplasm during the acute phase of infection. One of the most important findings about LAT is that it is partially antisense to the coding region encompassing the ICPO gene. The LR transcript is not restricted to HSV-1, but has been detected in swine latently infected with pseudorabies virus (PRV) [30], BHV [31, 32], and HSV-2 [Tenser, unpubl. data]. The two potentially polyadenylated species of PRV-specific LR RNAs detected in the trigeminal ganglia of these latently infected pigs were 2.0 and 0.95 kb. Rock et al. [33], using in situ hybridization and northern blot analyses, detected LR-RNAs in trigeminal ganglia of rabbits latently infected with HSV-1, thus confirming a transcriptionally active region in the vicinity of ICPO during the latency phase of infection. This finding also confirmed the presence of two major species (1.8–2.2 kb) LR-RNA, in trigeminal ganglia of infected rabbits [33]. Earlier work from the same laboratory detected bovine HSV-1 LR-RNA in trigeminal ganglia of latently infected rabbits [31, 32].

Thus far, the HSV LR transcripts are not unique to humans. They (LAT) have also been detected in experimentally infected mice [27, 34], rabbits [33] and probably guinea pigs [26] and are similar in size, location and direction of transcription as human LAT RNAs [35]. Deatly et al. [36] also demonstrated that mRNA from the IE region of HSV-1 genome is present in the trigeminal ganglia of latently infected mice, and further observed that the transcript is restricted to one region only in latently infected mouse trigeminal ganglia. Using probes directed to the IE genes ICP0, ICP4, ICP22 and ICP27 and ICP47, investigators found that only ICP0-directed probes gave positive hybridization signals for the presence of LAT. The positive LAT signal was detected by 1.6 kb *Sac*I subfragments of *Bam*HI PS restriction fragment and 2.6 and 6.8 kb *Sal*I subfragments of *Bam*HI B which were used as probes to separate the three IE region genes. The use of these probes gave 100% positive hybridization signals in the infected mice examined.

During HSV infection in cell culture, five IE genes were immediately transcribed to produce infected cell polypeptides ICP0, 4, 22, 27, and 47 [37]. Transcription of these genes requires no prior viral protein synthesis; however, the transcription of the subsequent class of genes, namely the early genes, requires the expression of the IE [38–45]. ICP4 and 27 are regulatory proteins essential for the regulation of the virus in cell culture; however, functional studies of ICP22 and 47 IE proteins show that deletion mutants of these genes are replication competent [41–44]. Despite its (ICP0) ability to transactivate alpha, beta and gamma genes, as defined by transient assays, its absence does not abrogate virus replication [46, 47]. Nevertheless, ICP0 can synergistically act with ICP4 to activate viral promoters [48–53]. A more detailed analysis of the signal from ICP0 sequences by Deatly et al. [36] and others [54, 55] show that the transcript being detected hybridized to *Bam*HI PS, B and E restriction fragments which encode ICP0 gene sequences.

The nature, structure and the source of the LAT RNAs became clearer when Spivack and Fraser [34] detected, by northern blot analysis, three transcripts from HSV-1 latently infected trigeminal ganglia of mice. Using the nick-translated HSV-1 (F strain) DNA probe corresponding to the *Bam*HI B restriction fragment, they could map LAT transcripts to a *Pst*I-*Mlu*I subfragment of *Bam*HI B. These mapped transcripts with measured sizes of 2.0, 1.5 and 1.45 kb were partially complementary and in the antisense orientation to ICP0. In all cases where a transcript was found in latently infected hosts, the hybridization was abolished in the presence of RNase but not DNase confirming earlier reports by Tenser et al. [26]. The HSV LAT transcript now is mapped to an area bordered by *Hpa*I restriction site to the left of *Bam*HI B fragment and to the right by *Mlu*I.

One or two possible species of LR RNA were detected in rabbits infected with HSV-1 (McKrae) through the ocular route of infection [31]. These LR-RNA were mapped to the area of ICP0 gene (IE-110) and ranged from 1.8 to 2.2 kb. In addition, these transcripts were partially complementary and antisense to ICP0. This finding shows that the route of entry of the virus does not influence the expression of LR-RNA transcripts. The corneal route of infection was also used in mice, guinea pigs and rabbits [26, 56].

In human trigeminal ganglia recovered at autopsy from 24 patients with no known history of herpesvirus infection, it was demonstrated that 72% of ganglionic neuronal extracts hybridized to an ^{35}S-labeled LAT-specific single-stranded probe, and the signal was localized primarily in the nucleus of the nerve cell [57, 58].

The presence of virus-specific RNA, which partially hybridized to the ICP0 gene region, also corresponds to the significantly elevated herpes-specific neutralizing antibodies in the patients [59, 60]. In a related study, Coren et al. [58] demonstrate that during varicella-zoster virus (VZV) infection of neuronal and non-neuronal cells, all VZV genes were expressed as detected by hybridization when ganglia was probed with several parts of the viral genome. In contrast to HSV infection where, during the latent phase of infection, few genes if any are expressed and the hybridization signal has been limited thus far to neurons [61]. In another study of human trigeminal ganglia, two abundant transcripts (1.85 and 1.35 kb) were detected in 9 of 17 individuals by northern (RNA) blot analysis utilizing a probe spanning the *Bam*HI PS region [62].

With the finding that a virus-specific mRNA is being transcribed in ganglionic neuronal cells in infected humans, Stevens et al. [63] further show that the presence of LAT corresponds to seropositivity to HSV antibody. This gives credence to the earlier report by Croen et al. [58], where seronegativity to HSV antibody resulted in lack of expression of LAT in trigeminal ganglia of autopsy patients. These findings further support the pre-

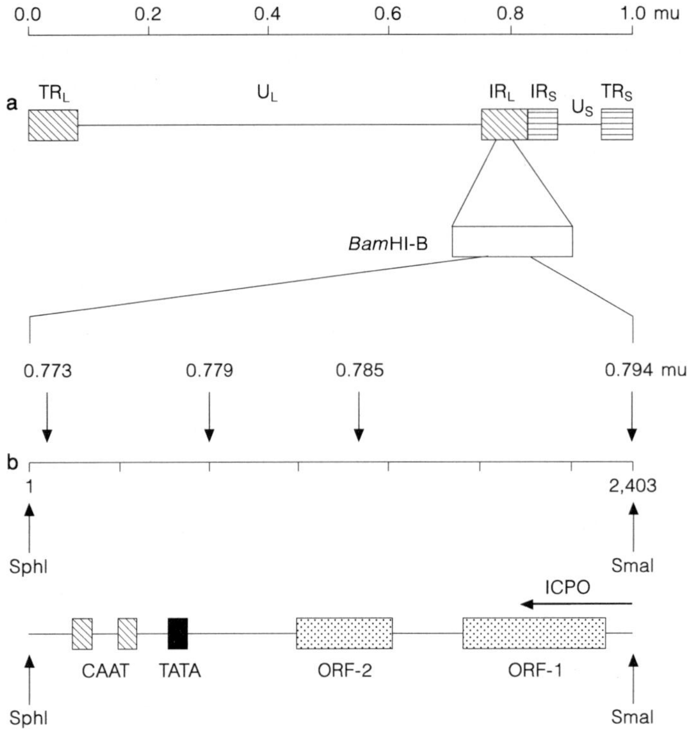

Fig. 1. The physical structure of LAT of HSV. **a** The HSV genome depicting long and small terminal and internal repeats, and unique long and small sequences. **b** The *Bam*HI-B subfragment showing nucleotide positions based on HSV-1 KOS (M) [64]. Some of the pertinent features of LAT transcript as identified by physical mapping of LAT in neurons include: CAAT ▧; TATA ■; and ORF-1 and ORF-2 [64].

mise that latency, as an inactive pathogenic process, is not entirely correct. Experimental evidence indicates that LAT partially overlaps the 3′ and of ICP0 and the opposite transcriptional polarity to the ICP0 gene in all human and murine model systems proposed so far.

Physical Structure of LAT

Physical characterization of LAT reveals 2–3 species spliced from a larger molecule depending on the system and techniques used (fig. 1). Specifically, Wagner et al. [64] have characterized extensively the physical nature of LAT from HSV-1 [McKrae or KOS (M)] infected rabbit and mice and found two species of LAT of sizes 2.1–2.2 and 0.73 kb. The small transcript which has a 730-bp intron is expressed colinearly with the larger. They also speculate that both the virus strain and the type of host are important in latency in maintaining the processing or stability of the spliced LAT transcripts. Additionally, Wagner et al. [65] did not find polyadenylated transcripts as reported by others [27, 66, 67]. Wagner et al. [64] provided the full nucleotide sequence of LAT from HSV-1 (KOS)-infected murine sensory nerve ganglia. The full sequence is published elsewhere [64]; howeve, the sequence covers the distance between the *Sph*I site to the left of the *Kpn*I site at 0.783 mu of HSV-1 genome and extends to the *Sma*I site 660 bases to the right of the *Sal*I site at 0.790 mu. There are two possible CAAT sequences at 108–110 and 145–150 and a possible TATA box beginning at nucleotide 171–179. There also is a CAP site at nucleotide 195, and there are characteristic groups of pyrimidines at nucleotide 18–45, 69–109 and 114–137. Other features of the sequence include 2 LAT open reading frames (ORFs) on at nucleotide 625–831 and the other at 1,160–2,074 in addition to ICP0 ORF at 1,720 in the opposite strand. Wechsler et al. [67, 68] have determined that the two ORFs should encode products of 12 and 36 kD for ORF-1 and ORF-2 with corresponding start codons at 1,028 and 958, respectively; however, the shorter LAT ORF is not conserved between HSV-1 strains. In support of the existence of differentially spiced species of LAT, Wechsler et al. [67] used ^{32}P-labeled genomic DNA restriction fragments and synthetic oligonucleotides as probes to analyze LAT in trigeminal ganglia of rabbits.

In a related study Wechsler et al. [67] modified previous findings with regard to the structure of the LR gene. New evidence indicates that the 2-kb LR transcript has two ORFs and no introns, but the presence of a novel upstream TATA box (–688 to –664) which functions as a promoter in CAT assays has been observed [Wechsler, unpubl. data].

This LAT promoter is functionally specific for neuronal cells. A single intron, in addition to the two ORFs, also has been identified in the 1.3–1.5 kb LR transcript. Characteristics of these LRs include a faint upstream and downstream transcription (by in situ hybridization) of both 2.0 kb and 1.3–1.5 kb LR genes. Futher evidence suggests that the two stable LR transcripts may result from the processing of an unstable larger 8.3-kb precursor transcript. The mechanisms leading to the formation of the two stable LRs are not understood [68] (fig. 2).

In an attempt to define transcriptional regulatory elements for LAT, Dobson et al. [69] concludes that the TATA box at 171–179 is a probable promoter element. Using a recombinant HSV-1, they found that the LAT TATA box elements were able to express rabbit beta-globulin when the globulin gene was placed downstream of the TATA box. Furthermore, removal of the TATA box sequences resulted in the lack of expression of LAT in the latently infected host. The location of the LAT promoter indicates that the mRNA upstream is degraded after transcription. From current information on LAT, the following statements were made by Dobson et al. [69]: (i) LAT is probably regulated by conventional *Pol*II promoter elements; (ii) stable LAT is processed from a primary, unstable larger transcript thatt is polyadenylated in acute infection and not in latent infection; (iii) LATs flanking splicing sequences coupled with its non-polyadenylated nuclear transcripts suggest that LAT may be an intron.

Comparison of various LAT from different strains of HSV-1 shows that in strain F, 17 syn$^+$ and KOS there are two possible ORF common to all, but the shorter one is not conserved among HSV-1 strains. In addition, there are three to four SP1-binding sites at –887 and –589, a CAAT element at –817 and TATA box at –587 all indicating a transcriptional promoter but no consensus promoter sequences [67, 68] and ORF-1 and ORF-2

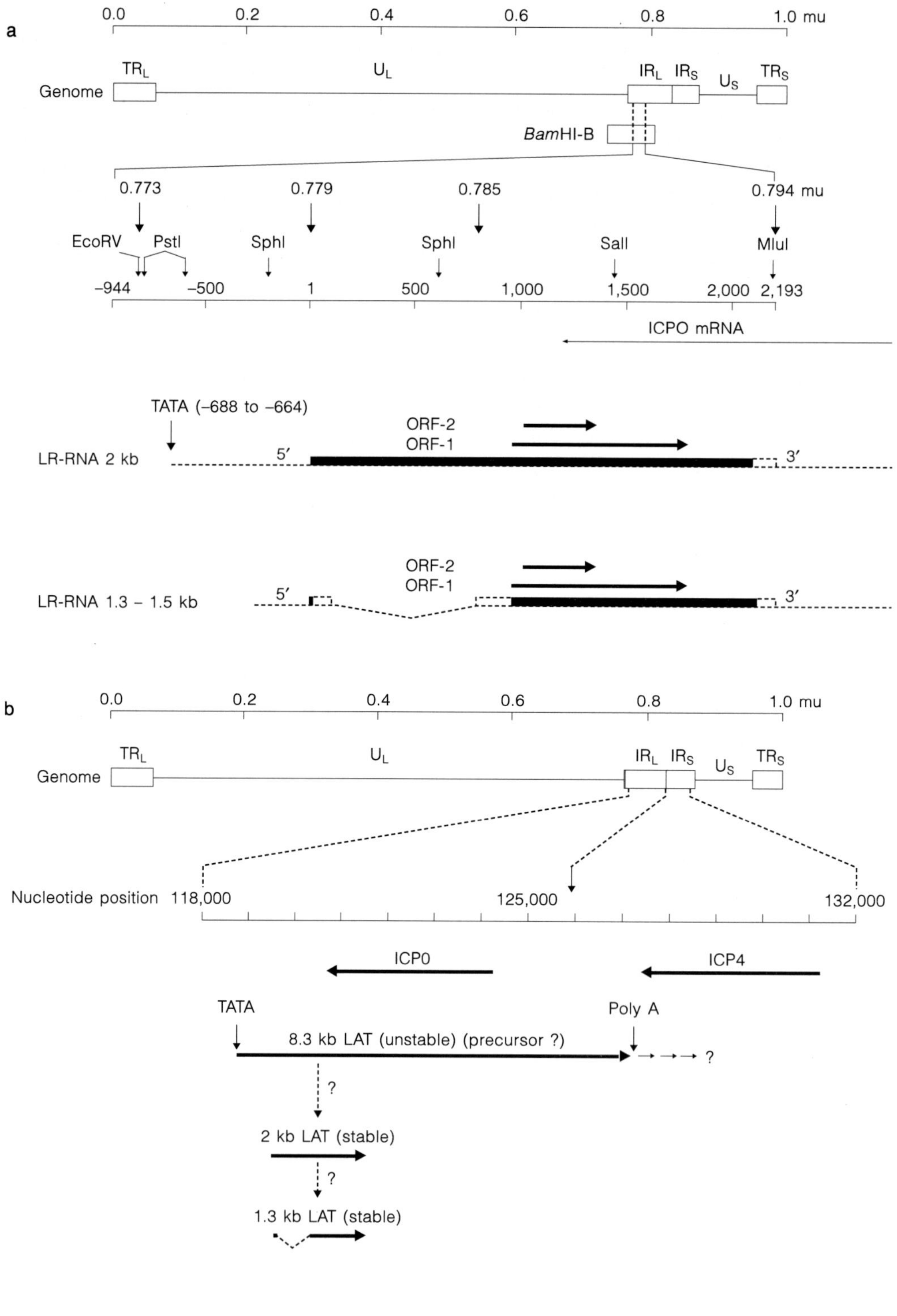
a
0.0
0.2
0.4
0.6
0.8
1.0 mu
Genome
TRL
UL
IRL
IRS
US
TRS
BamHI-B
0.773
0.779
0.785
0.794 mu
EcoRV
PstI
SphI
SphI
SalI
MluI
–944
–500
1
500
1,000
1,500
2,000
2,193
ICPO mRNA
TATA (–688 to –664)
LR-RNA 2 kb
5′
3′
ORF-2
ORF-1
LR-RNA 1.3 – 1.5 kb
b
Nucleotide position
118,000
125,000
132,000
ICP0
ICP4
TATA
Poly A
8.3 kb LAT (unstable) (precursor ?)
?
2 kb LAT (stable)
1.3 kb LAT (stable)

make no detectable proteins by current available techniques [68, 69].

Possible Functions of LAT

The function and role of LAT in the establishment, maintenance and reactivation of HSV latent infection are not known. For instance, LAT was reported to be unnecessary for the establishment of latency [70]. In an attempt to explain the tissue specificity of HSV reactivation from latency, Deatly et al. [71] used explant reactivation assays in addition to in situ hybridization to explain why explants from latently infected peripheral nervous system (PNS) are reactivatable and explants from the CNS are not. LAT was expressed by both, and it was not apparent that reactivation of HSV from latency was dependent on the extent of LAT genome transcription. However, this study does not rule out the possible involvement of LAT in reactivation of latent herpesvirus. This report concludes that host differences in CNS and PNS tissue specificity may determine ability of latent HSV-1 to reactivate. Spivack and Fraser [72] attempted to make the connection between transcription of LAT and HSV-1 reactivation making the following observations: (i) temporal expression of LAT genes at the acute phase (productively infected tissue culture) of infection is different from the expression of other HSV-1 genes during replication; (ii) there is a twof old decrease in LAT expression during reactivation, a state of infection when there is increased DNA synthesis and recoverable infectious virus; (iii) based on blocking of reactivation by phosphonoacetic acid (PPA) or novobiocin, LAT expression is an early event before entry of latent virus into the replication cycle. The 2.0 kb is detected in tissue and the expression of LAT appears to be cell or tissue-type specific [31–33].

Fig. 2. The structure of LR transcript gene fragment. **a** The upper portion denotes HSV-1 genomic organization in map units (mu). The expanded region indicates nucleotide position relative to the entire HSV-1 DNA sequence and relative to the 5′-end (+1) of the stable 2- and 1.3-kb LATs. The location of the TATA box sequences and of the 2- and 1.3-kb LAT are shown for reference. The faint transcript from up- and downstream RNA of LAT gene is shown in dashed lines while the LAT transcript is shown in dark rectangles. **b** The location of the large possibly unstable 8.3-kb LAT that may be the precursor of the two stable LATs. The exact 3′-end is not clear; however, the sequence of processing of the two LATs is shown [67, 68, personal commun.] (figure supplied by Dr. Wechsler).

In a more elaborate experiment involving the use of deletion mutant HFEM, it was found that LAT is not an IE gene [72]. The expression of early and late genes is known to require the expression of IE [37, 40, 47, 48, 50–55]. However, LAT expression is not dependent on the expression of IE genes. This observation came from a metabolic inhibitor and strand-specific hybridization studies [72]. Since LAT may function more in latency than in a replication cycle, the authors propose that LAT RNAs constitute a new class of genes which they call lambda (λ).

The function or role of LAT RNAs during or in latency is uncertain. However, by process of elimination LAT was reported to be nonessential for the establishment of latent infection [73]. In this report, HSV-1 strain 17 syn^+ and variant 1,704 with deletion of 3.8 and 1.2 kb in IR_L and TR_L, respectively, were used to infect mice. It was demonstrated that the variant replicated in the trigeminal ganglia of infected mice as efficiently as the wild-type 17 syn$^+$. Nevertheless, the reactivation of the 1,704 mutants was relatively prolonged compared to the wild-type 17 syn$^+$. The 17 syn$^+$ wild-type virus produced LAT transcripts, but the mutant 1,704 did not as determined by either in situ hybridization or northern blot analyses. Leib et al. [74], in an attempt to determine the function of LAT, found that LAT-deleted mutants reactivate from latency with reduced frequency. Additionally, marker-rescue and transfection studies show that sequences involved in transcription of LAT are nonessential for the establishment of or reactivation from latency, despite the infrequency of reactivation in deletion mutants [75].

A HSV-1 DNA fragment *Bam*HI-B was reported to be associated with the phenotype of intraperitoneal pathogenicity [76–79]. This finding raised the question of whether or not LAT is associated with the pathogenicity of HSV infection. Others, using a host of wild-type and mutant HSV viruses, have demonstrated that DNA sequences in the area of the *Bam*HI B restriction fragment are involved in the complex mechanism of the pathogenesis of latent HSV infection [79].

Several groups [19, 20, 26] investigated the relationship between LAT and TK in TK mutants and wild-type HSV-1. Tenser et al. [26] found that LAT is present in the sensory ganglia of the nervous system of mice after infection with HSV-1 TK$^-$ mutant. The mutant can establish latency, but no reactivatable virus was found in sensory ganglion neuron after infection of mice with the TK$^-$ mutant. Similarly, Leist et al. [20] observed that the HSV-1 variant C239 (TK$^-$) can establish latency at levels slightly below the wild-type HSV-1 (KOS) and the TK$^-$ rescued variant, but the C239 (TK$^-$) variant was not reactivatable when cultured in vitro. They suggested that if LAT is equated with the presence of latent HSV infection, then TK$^-$ mutants can establish latency but may be defective in reactivation.

One of the many possible functions for LAT is that the transcript may be translated into proteins which in turn will modulate ICP0 genes [33, 34, 80, 81]. Others [29, 82] suggest that the putative LAT protein may initiate a lytic cycle in virus-infected cells. However, due to nuclear retention of the transcript, translation will be aborted, and subsequent termination of cell lysis will occur in the infected host. The problem with this hypothesis is that no LAT-encoded proteins have been found in latently infected neurons. Recently, data from Hill et al. [56] indicate that HSV latent phase transcription may facilitate in vivo reactivation of the virus from latency. In mice, the HSV-1 variant X10-13 produced no LAT, but it established latency and produced LAT minus progeny in explanted cultures and cocultivated sensory ganglionic neural cultures. When rabbits were infected through either cornea or conjunctiva, X10-13 again was able to establish latent infection in trigeminal ganglia and subsequently became reactivatable. However, XC-20 variant derivative of rescued X10-13, which is LAT positive, reactivated significantly at a higher level than X10-13. Based on this and other findings, the authors conclude that latent phase transcription of HSV-1 facilitates ganglionic reactivation.

Due to the nuclear localization of LAT, one postulate for its function has been that LAT serves as a trans-acting or *cis*-acting factor that can physically prevent ICP0 transcription by binding on the opposite strand of the same stretch of DNA. This will effectively block ICP0 gene transcription and result in subsequent blockage of beta- and gamma-genes transcription, which depends on alpha-gene transcription in the HSV gene expression cascade.

However, Ho and Mocarski [21] conclude that LAT is not involved in any antisense regulatory mechanism, nor was LAT-encoded protein involved in the establishment or maintenance of latency in mouse. These conclusions were based on data from recombinant virus HSV-1 RH142 studies in which both LAT promoters of HSV-1 did not induce the production of any detectable LAT during latent or productive infection in cells. However, the β-galactoside Lac-Z reporter gene was expressed in sensory neurons in latently infected mice when placed downstream of LAT promoters. This [21] and other observations [31, 32, 83] indicate that the cell or tissue-type specificity of the kinetics of LAT expression differs from other HSV-1 genes [31, 32, 83]. For instance, Wagner et al. [65] have shown that the strain of virus and the type of host (mouse, human or rabbit) influence the splicing products. More recently, Batchelor and O'Hare [83] confirmed and extended virus strain and tissue-type specificity as influencing factors in the LAT expression kinetics in HeLa and neuroblastoma (IMR-32) cells.

Conclusions

In conclusion, during the latent phase of HSV infection, there is virus-specific transcription of the virus genome into mRNA called LAT. There are two or possibly three LAT transcripts found in all the systems studied, including animals and humans. The consensus sizes [64, 65, 67, 68] of the two LAT transcripts are 2.0 and 1.3–1.45 kb, and are transcribed in an antisense orientation to the IE gene, ICP0. The area encoding the LAT transcript has been mapped to the *Bam*HI B restriction fragment (0.738–0.807 mu) of the HSV-1 genome. The exact function of these transcripts is not known. However, it is known that they are not essential for the establishment of and reactivation from latency. With no known product (i.e. protein) assigned to LAT transcripts, the possibility of LAT as a regulatory factor in the complex milieu of events leading to HSV latency following the acute infection is not illogical. Most of the evidence suggests that LAT may be involved in the maintenance of HSV latency. However, more recent findings indicate that latent phase transcription may facilitate in vivo reactivation. Another possible role is that the transcripts function as *cis*- and/or trans-acting factors, in modulating the expression of at least IE and early gene expression, and are required for production of infectious virus. However, Ho and Mocarski [21] argue against any antisense regulatory mechanism of LAT in the regulation of viral gene expression or any role of LAT-encoded protein (nondetected) during the establishment or maintenance of latency. Nevertheless, LAT is not involved in the establishment [70, 73] or reactivation [74, 75] of latent HSV.

Acknowledgments

We are grateful to Dr. Richard B. Tenser for his critical review and helpful suggestions. We thank Ann Viozzi for the editorial work and Elaine Neidigh for typing the manuscript. This study was supported in part by National Cancer Institute Grants CA27503 and CA34479 and by BRSG Grant S07 RR05680-21 awarded by the Biomedical Research Support Grant Program, Division of Research Resources, NIH.

References

1 Cushing H: The surgical aspects of major neuralgia of the trigeminal nerve: A report of 20 cases of operation on the Gasserian ganglion, with anatomic and physiologic notes on the consequences of its removal. JAMA 1905;44:1002–1008.
2 Goodpasture EW: Herpetic infections with special reference to involvement of the nervous system. Medicine 1929;8:223–224.
3 Doerr R: Herpes febrilis; in Doerr R, Hallaver C (eds): Der Virus-forschung. Vienna, Springer, 1938, vol 1, pp 41–45.
4 Roizman B: An inquiry into the mechanisms of recurrent herpes infections in man; in Pollard M (ed): Perspectives in Virology. New York, Harper & Row, 1966, vol 4, pp 283–304.
5 Klein RJ: Initiation and maintenance of latent herpes simplex virus infection: The paradox of perpetual immobility and continuous movement. Rev Infect Dis 1985;7:21–30.
6 Roizman B, Sears AE: An inquiry into the mechanisms of herpes simplex virus latency. Ann Rev Microbiol 1987;41:543–571.
7 Baichwal VR, Sugden B: Latency comes of age for herpesviruses. Cell 1988;52:787–789.
8 Fraser NW, Deatly AM, Mellerick DM, McDougall JK, Spivack JG: Molecular biology of latent HSV-1; in Lopez C, Roizman B (eds): Human Herpesvirus Infection: Pathogenesis, Diagnosis, and Treatment. New York, Raven Press, 1986, pp 39–54.
9 Hill TJ: Herpes simplex virus latency; in Roizman B (ed): The Herpesviruses. New York, Plenum Press, 1985, vol 4, pp 175–240.
10 Stevens JG, Cook ML: Latent herpes simplex virus in spinal ganglia of mice. Science 1971; 173:843–845.
11 Cook ML, Bastone VB, Stevens JG: Evidence that neurons harbor latent herpes simplex virus. Infect Immun 1974;9:946–951.
12 McLennan JL, Darby G: Herpes simplex virus latency: The cellular location of virus in dorsal root ganglia and the fate of the infected cell following virus activation. J Gen Virol 1980;51: 233–243.
13 Deshmane SL, Fraser NW: During latency herpes simplex virus type 1 DNA is associated with nucleosomes in a chromatin structure. J Virol 1989; 63:943–947.
14 Muggeridge MI, Fraser NW: Chromosomal organization of the herpes simplex virus genome during acute infection of the mouse central nervous system. J Virol 1986;59:764–767.
15 Mellerick DM, Fraser NW: Physical state of the latent herpes simplex virus genome in a mouse model system: Evidence suggesting an episomal state. Virology 1987;158:265–275.
16 Rock DL, Fraser NW: Latent herpes simplex virus type 1 DNA contains two copies of the virion DNA joint region. J Virol 1985;55:849–852.
17 Efstathiou S, Minson AC, Field HJ, Anderson JR, Wildy P: Detection of herpes simplex virus-specific DNA sequences in latently infected mice and in humans. J Virol 1986;57:446–455.
18 Tenser RB, Hay KA, Edris WA: Latency-associated transcript but not reactivatable virus is present in sensory ganglion neurons after inoculation of thymidine kinase-negative mutants of herpes simplex virus type 1. J Virol 1989;63: 2861–2865.
19 Coen DM, Kosz-Vnenchak M, Jacobson JG, Leib DA, Bogard CL, Schaffer PA, Tyler KL, Knipe DM: Thymidine kinase-negative herpes simplex virus mutants establish latency in mouse trigeminal ganglia but do not reactivate. Proc Natl Acad Sci USA 1989;86:4736–4740.
20 Leist TP, Sandri-Goldin RM, Stevens JG: Latent infections in spinal ganglia with thymidine kinase-deficient herpes simplex virus. J Virol 1989;63:4976–4978.
21 Ho DY, Mocarski ES: Herpes simplex virus latent RNA (LAT) is not required for latent infection in mouse. Proc Natl Acad Sci USA 1989;86:7596–7600.
22 Galloway DA, Fenoglio C, Shevchuk M, McDougall JK: Detection of herpes simples RNA in human sensory ganglia. Virology 1979;95: 265–268.
23 Galloway DA, Fenoglio CM, McDougall JK: Limited transcription of the herpes simplex virus genome when latent in human sensory ganglia. J Virol 1982;41:686–691.
24 Steiner I, Spivack JG, Jackson A, Lavi E, Fraser NW: Effects of lipofuscin on in situ hybridization in human neuronal tissue. J Virol Method 1989; 24:1–10.
25 Stroop WG, Rock DL, Fraser NW: Localization of herpes simplex virus in the trigeminal and olfactory system of the mouse central nervous sys-

tem during acute and latent infection by in situ hybridization. Lab Invest 1984;51:27–38.
26 Tenser RB, Dawson M, Ressel SJ, Dunstan ME: Detection of herpes simplex virus mRNA in latently infected trigeminal ganglion neurons by in situ hybridization. Ann Neurol 1982;11:285–291.
27 Puga A, Notkins AL: Continued expression of a poly(A)$^+$ transcript of herpes simplex virus type 1 in trigeminal ganglia of latent infected mice. J Virol 1987;61:1700–1703.
28 Gelman IH, Silverstein S: Identification of immediate early genes from herpes simplex virus that transactivate the virus thymidine kinase gene. Proc Natl Acad Sci USA 1985;82:5265–5269.
29 Stevens JG, Wagner EK, Devi-Rao GB, Cook ML, Feldman LT: RNA complementary to a herpesvirus alpha gene mRNA is prominent in latently infected neurons. Science 1987;235:1056–1059.
30 Cheung AK: Detection of pseudorabies virus transcripts in trigeminal ganglia of latently infected swine. J Virol 1989;63:2908–2913.
31 Rock DL, Beam SL, Mayfield JE: Mapping bovine herpesvirus type 1 latency-related RNA in trigeminal ganglia of latently infected rabbits. J Virol 1987 ;61:3827–3831.
32 Rock DL, Hagemoser WA, Osorio FA, Reed DE: Detection of bovine herpesvirus type 1 RNA in trigeminal ganglia of latently infected rabbits by in situ hybridization. J Gen Virol 1986;67:2515–2520.
33 Rock DL, Nesburn AB, Ghiasi H, Ong J, Lewis TL, Lokensgard JR, Wechsler SL: Detection of latency-related viral RNAs in trigeminal ganglia of rabbits latently infected with herpes simplex virus type 1. J Virol 1987;61:3820–3826.
34 Spivack JG, Fraser NW: Detection of herpes simplex virus type 1 transcripts during latent infection in mice. J Virol 1987;61:3841–3847.
35 Steiner I, Spivack JG, O'Boyle II DR, Lavi E, Fraser NW: Latent herpes simples virus type 1 transcription in human trigeminal ganglia. J Virol 1988;62:3493–3496.
36 Deatly AM, Spivack JG, Lavi E, Fraser NW: RNA from an immediate early region of the type 1 herpes simplex virus genome is present in the trigeminal ganglia of latently infected mice. Proc Natl Acad Sci USA 1987;84:3204–3208.
37 Pereira L, Wolff MH, Fenwick M, Roizman B: Regulation of herpesvirus macromolecular synthesis. V. Properties of alpha polypeptides made in HSV-1 and HSV-2 infected cells. Virology 1973;77:733–749.
38 Clements JB, Watson RJ, Wilkie NM: Temporal regulation of herpes simplex virus type 1 transcription: Location of transcripts on the viral genome. Cell 1977;12:275–285.
39 Dixon RAF, Schaffer PA: Feine-structure mapping and functional analysis of temperature-sensitive mutants in the gene encoding the herpes simplex virus type 1 immediate early protein VP175. J Virol 1980;36:189–203.
40 Honess RW, Roizman B: Regulation of herpesvirus macromolecular synthesis: sequential transition of polypeptide snythesis requires functional viral polypeptides. Proc Natl Acad Sci USA 1975;72:1276–1280.
41 Smith CA, Marchetti ME, Edmonson P, Schaffer PA: Herpes simplex virus type 2 mutants with deletions in the intergenic region between ICP4 and ICP22/47: Identification of nonessential *cis*-acting elements in the context of the viral genome. J Virol 1989;63:2036–2047.
42 DeLuca NA, McCarthy A, Schaffer PA: Location and characterization of deletion mutants of herpes simplex virus type 1 in the gene encoding immediate-early regulatory proteins ICP4. J Virol 1985;50:538–570.
43 McCarthy AM, McMahan L, Schaffer PA: Herpes simplex virus type 1 ICP27 deletion mutants exhibit altered patterns of transcription and are DNA deficient. J Virol 1989;63:18–27.
44 Rice SA, Su L, Knipe DM: Herpes simplex virus alpha protein ICP27 possesses separate positive and negative regulatory activities. J Virol 1989;63:3399–3407.
45 Preston CM: Control of herpes simplex virus type 1 mRNA synthesis in cells infected with wild-type virus or the temperature-sensitive mutant tsK. J Virol 1979;29:275–284.
46 DeLuca NA, Schaffer PA: Activation of immediate-early, early, and late promoters by temperature-sensitive and wild-type forms of herpes simplex virus type 1 protein ICP4. Mol Cell Biol 1985;5:1997–2008.
47 Everett RD: The products of herpes simplex virus type 1 (HSV-1) immediate early genes 1, 2 and 3 can activate HSV-1 gene expression in *trans*. J Gen Virol 1986;67:2507–2513.
48 Everett RD: Transactivation of transcription by

herpesvirus products: requirement for two HSV-1 immediate-early polypeptides for maximum activity. EMBO J 1984;3:3135–3141.

49 Mavromara-Nazos P, Silver S, Hubenthal-Voss J, McKnight JLC, Roizman B: Regulation of herpes simplex virus 1 genes: Alpha gene sequence requirements for transient induction of indicator genes regulated by beta or late (gamma$_2$) promoters. Virology 1986;149:152–164.

50 O'Hare P, Hayward GS: Evidence for a direct role for both the 175,000 and 110,000-molecular-weight immediate-early proteins of herpes simplex virus in the transactivation of delayed-early promoters. J Virol 1985;53:751–760.

51 Quinlan MP, Knipe DM: Stimulation of expression of a herpes simplex virus DNA-binding protein by two viral functions. Mol Cell Biol 1985; 5:957–963.

52 Sacks WR, Greene CC, Aschman DP, Schaffer PA: Herpes simplex virus type 1 ICP27 is an essential regulatory protein. J Virol 1985;55:796–805.

53 Stow ND, Stow EC: Isolation and characterization of a herpes simplex virus type 1 mutant containing a deletion within the gene encoding the immediate early polypeptide Vmw110. J Gen Virol 1986;67:2571–2585.

54 Clements JB, McLauchlan J, McGeoch OJ: Orientation of herpes simplex virus type 1 immediate early mRNAs. Nucl Acid Res 1979;7:77–91.

55 Mackem S, Roizman B: Regulation of herpes virus macromolecular synthesis: Transcription-initiation sites and domains of alpha genes. Proc Natl Acad Sci USA 1980;77:7122–7126.

56 Hill JM, Sedarati F, Javier RT, Wagner EK, Stevens JG: Herpes simplex virus latent phase transcription facilitates in vivo reactivation. Virology 1990;174:117–125.

57 Gordon YJ, Johnson B, Romanowski E, Araullo-Cruz T: RNA complementary to herpes simplex virus type 1 ICP0 gene demonstrated in neurons of human trigeminal ganglia. J Virol 1988;62: 1832–1835.

58 Croen KD, Ostrove JM, Dragovic LJ, Smialek JE, Straus SE: Latent herpes simples virus in human trigeminal ganglia. Detection of an immediate early gene 'anti-sense' transcript in situ hybridization. N Engl J Med 1987;317:1427–1432.

59 Hyman RW, Ecker JR, Tenser RB: Varicella-zoster virus RNA in human trigeminal ganglia. Lancet 1983;ii:814–816.

60 Gilden DH, Rozenman Y, Murray R, Delvin M, Vafai A: Detection of varicella-zoster virus nucleic acid in neurons of normal human thoracic ganglia. Ann Neurol 1987;22:377–380.

61 Croen KD, Ostrove JM, Dragovic LJ, Straus SE: Patterns of gene expression and sites of latency in human nerve ganglia are different for varicella-zoster and herpes simplex viruses. Proc Natl Acad Sci USA 1988;85:9773–9777.

62 Krause PR, Croen KD, Straus SE, Ostrove JM: Detection and preliminary characterization of herpes simplex virus type 1 transcripts in latently infected human trigeminal ganglia. J Virol 1988; 62:4819–4823.

63 Stevens JG, Haarr L, Porter DD, Cook ML, Wagner EK: Prominence of the herpes simplex virus latency-associated transcript in trigeminal ganglia from seropositive humans. J Infect Dis 1988;158:117–123.

64 Wagner EK, Devi-Rao G, Feldman LT, Dobson AT, Zhang Y-F, Flanagan WM, Stevens JG: Physical characterization of the herpes simplex virus latency-associated transcript in neurons. J Virol 1988;62:1194–1202.

65 Wagner EK, Flanagan WM, Devi-Rao G, Zhang Y-F, Hill JM, Anderson KP, Stevens JG: The herpes simplex virus latency-associated transcript is spliced during the latent phase of infection. J Virol 1988;62:4577–4585.

66 Spivack JG, Fraser NW: Expression of herpes simplex virus type 1 latency-associated transcript in trigeminal ganglia of mice during acute infection and reactivation of latent infection. J Virol 1988;62:1479–1485.

67 Wechsler SL, Nesburn AB, Zwaagstra J, Ghiasi H: Sequence of the latency-related gene of herpes simplex virus type 1. Virology 1989;168:168–172.

68 Wechsler SL, Nesburn AB, Watson R, Slanina SM, Ghiasi H: Fine mapping of the latency-related gene of herpes simplex virus type 1: Alternative splicing produces distinct latency-related RNAs containing open reading frames. J Virol 1988;62:4051–4058.

69 Dobson AT, Sederati F, Devi-Rao G, Flanagan WM, Farrell MJ, Stevens JG, Wagner EK, Feldman LT: Identification of the latency-associated transcript promoter by expression of rabbit beta-globin mRNA in mouse sensory nerve ganglia latently infected with a recombinant herpes simplex virus. J Virol 1989;63:3844–3851.

70 Javier RT, Stevens JG, Dissette VB, Wagner EK: A herpes simplex virus transcript abundant in latently infected neurons is dispensable for establishment of the latent state. Virology 1988;166: 254–257.
71 Deatly AM, Spivack JG, Lavi E, O'Boyle DR II, Fraser NW: Latent herpes simples virus type 1 transcripts in peripheral and central nervous system tissues of mice map to similar regions of the viral genome. J Virol 1988;62:749–756.
72 Spivack JG, Fraser NW: Expression of herpes simplex virus type 1 latency-associated transcripts and transcripts affected by the deletion in avirulent mutant NFEM: Evidence for a new class of HSV-1 genes. J Virol 1988;62:3281–3287.
73 Steiner I, Spivack JG, Lirette RP, Brown SM, MacLean AR, Subak-Sharpe JH, Fraser NW: Herpes simplex virus type 1 latency-associated transcripts are evidently not essential for latent infection. EMBO J 1989;8:505–511.
74 Leib DA, Coen DM, Bogard CL, Hicks KA, Yager DR, Knipe DM, Tyler KL, Schaffer PA: Immediate-early regulatory gene mutants define different stages in the establishment and reactivation of herpes simplex virus latency. J Virol 1989;63: 759–768.
75 Leib DA, Bogard CL, Kosz-Vnenchak M, Hicks KA, Coen DM, Knipe DM, Schaffer PA: A deletion mutant of the latency-associated transcript of herpes simplex virus type 1 reactivates from the latent state with reduced frequency. J Virol 1989;63:2893–2900.
76 Rosen A, Darai G: Mapping of the deletion in the genome HSV-1 strain HFEM responsible for its avirulent phenotype. Med Microbiol Immunol 1985;173:329–343.
77 Becker Y, Hadar J, Tabor E, Ben-Hur T, Raibstein I, Rosen A, Darai G: A sequence in *HpaI* P fragment of herpes simplex virus-1 DNA determines intraperitoneal virulence in mice. Virology 1986; 149:255–259.
78 Ben-Hur T, Moyal M, Rosen-Wolff A, Darai G, Becker Y: Characterization of RNA transcripts from herpes simplex virus-1 DNA fragment *Bam*HI B. Virology 1989;169:1–8.
79 Rosen-Wolff A, Scholz J, Darai G: Organotropism of latent herpes simplex virus type 1 is correlated to the presence of a 1.5 kb RNA transcript mapped within the *Bam*HI DNA fragment B (0.738–0.809 map units). Virus Res 1989;12:43–52.
80 Green PJ, Pines O, Inouye M: The role of antisense RNA in gene regulation. Ann Rev Biochem 1986;55:569–597.
81 Kim SK, Wold BJ: Stable reduction of thymidine kinase activity in cells expressing high levels of anti-sense RNA. Cell 1985;42:129–138.
82 Perry LJ, Rixon FJ, Everett RD, Frame MC, McGeoch DJ: Characterization of the IE110 gene of herpes simplex virus type 1. J Gen Virol 1986;67:2365–2380.
83 Batchelor AH, O'Hare P: Regulation and cell-type-specific activity of a promoter located upstream of the latency-associated transcript of herpes simplex virus type 1. J Virol 1990;64: 3269–3279.

Forthcoming Papers

Stimulation of Measles Virus Replication by Cyclic Guanosine Monophosphate
Robbins, S.J.

Homologous Recombination of a Plasmid Containing the SV40 Early Region in Rabbit Cells
Legrand, A.; Nachtigal, M.

Myristylation of the Envelope Glycoprotein of Vesicular Stomatitis Virus
Chen, S.S.-L.

Structural Comparison of the External Glycoproteins of Human Immunodeficiency Virus Simian Immunodeficiency Virus
Lüke, W.; Fendrich, C.; Sprenger, R.; Rietschel, J.; Hunsmann, G.

A Replication-Defective Variant of Sabin 3 Poliovirus
Tershak, D.R.; Allegretto, K.D.

Effects of Poliovirus Replication of Undifferentiated and Differentiated Monocytic U937 Cells: Comparative Studies with Human Macrophages
López-Guerrero, J.A.; Cabañas, C.; Bernabeu, C.; Fresno, M.; Alonso, M.A.

Antibody Reactivity to Deletion Mutants of the HIV-1 SF2 Envelope
Back, N.K.T.; Haigwood, N.L.; de Wolf, F.; de Jongh, B.M.; Goudsmit, J.

Extracellular Production of Mouse Interferon Beta by the *Bacillus subtilis* Alpha-Amylase Secretion Vectors: Antiviral Activity and Deduced NH_2-Terminal Amino Acid Sequences of the Secreted Proteins
Nakazawa, K.; Sasamoto, H.; Shiraki, Y.; Harada, S.; Yanagi, K.; Yamane, K.

Oligonucleotide Probes for the Specific Detection of the Wild Poliovirus Types 1 and 3 Endemic to Brazil
da Silva, E.E.; Pallansch, M.A.; Holloway, B.P.; Couto Oliveira, M.J.; Schatzmayr, H.G.; Kew, O.M.

Epstein-Barr Virus in Oropharyngeal and Nasopharyngeal Secretions of Patients with Nasopharyngeal Carcinoma and Control Subjects
Tsao, S.Y.; He, Y.; Cheng, P.M.N.; Ho, S.; Leung, S.F.; Shihman Chang, R.

Evidence of ssDNA in Tubulofilamentous Particles: Their Relationship to Scrapie-Associated Fibrils
Narang, H.K.